Nutrition, Genetics, and Cardiovascular Disease

Nutrition, Genetics, and Cardiovascular Disease

Editors

Marwan El Ghoch
Said El Shamieh

MDPI • Basel • Beijing • Wuhan • Barcelona • Belgrade • Manchester • Tokyo • Cluj • Tianjin

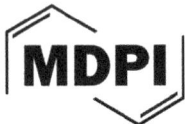

Editors

Marwan El Ghoch
Beirut Arab University
Lebanon

Said El Shamieh
Beirut Arab University
Lebanon

Editorial Office
MDPI
St. Alban-Anlage 66
4052 Basel, Switzerland

This is a reprint of articles from the Special Issue published online in the open access journal *Journal of Cardiovascular Development and Disease* (ISSN 2308-3425) (available at: https://www.mdpi.com/journal/jcdd/special_issues/cardiovascular_disease_nutrition).

For citation purposes, cite each article independently as indicated on the article page online and as indicated below:

LastName, A.A.; LastName, B.B.; LastName, C.C. Article Title. *Journal Name* **Year**, *Article Number, Page Range.*

ISBN 978-3-03943-240-0 (Hbk)
ISBN 978-3-03943-241-7 (PDF)

Contents

About the Editors

Marwan El Ghoch, MD earned a degree in Medicine and Surgery from the University of Bologna, Italy, and postgraduate studies in Clinical Nutrition from the University of Modena and Reggio Emilia, Italy. He is considered an expert on obesity and eating disorders treatments, and an established international leader in the study of body composition in eating disorders and obesity. He currently holds the role of head of the Department of Nutrition and Dietetics at Beirut Arab University in Lebanon. He is the author of more than 100 papers published in high-ranking peer-review journals in the field of medicine, human nutrition, and dietetics, and he is a member of the editorial of several scientific journals.

Said El Shamieh, Ph.D. is currently an associate professor of Human Genetics and Genomics at Beirut Arab University. Dr. Shamieh got an M.Sc. in Molecular, cellular, and Structural Biology, Université de Lorraine, France, then undertook a Ph.D. in Human Genetics at the same University. In 2012, he started a post-doctorate fellowship, Institut de la Vision, Sorbonne Universités, Pierre et Marie Curie, Paris, France. Dr. Shamieh's Research focuses on undergoing genotype–phenotype associations to identify genetic variants being implicated in cardiovascular disease risk factors and inherited retinal diseases. He published 50 international papers in journals; *American Journal of Human Genetics*, *Human Molecular Genetics*, and *Genes*. He is also a co-inventor of the patent WO2013093091. He currently serves as a reviewer for numerous journals such as *British Journal of Ophthalmology*, *Genes*, *Translational Vision Science and Technology*, *International Journal of Molecular Sciences*, *Clinica Chimica Acta*.

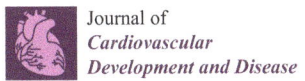

Journal of
Cardiovascular
Development and Disease

Editorial

Is There a Link Between Nutrition, Genetics, and Cardiovascular Disease?

Marwan El Ghoch [1],* and Said El Shamieh [2]

[1] Department of Nutrition and Dietetics, Faculty of Health Sciences, Beirut Arab University,
P.O. Box 11-5020 Riad El Solh, Beirut 11072809, Lebanon
[2] Department of Medical Laboratory Technology, Faculty of Health Sciences, Beirut Arab University,
P.O. Box 11-5020 Riad El Solh, Beirut 11072809, Lebanon; s.elshamieh@bau.edu.lb
* Correspondence: m.ghoch@bau.edu.lb

Received: 26 August 2020; Accepted: 26 August 2020; Published: 27 August 2020

Cardiovascular diseases (CVDs) are a group of disorders that mainly include coronary, cerebrovascular and rheumatic heart diseases [1]. CVDs are the primary cause of death worldwide, and genetic and environmental factors seem to play a determinant role in this [1]. In fact, cardiovascular diseases are strongly associated with certain lifestyle factors (i.e., diet and physical inactivity) [2,3] and nutrition-related diseases (i.e., obesity and type 2 diabetes) [4]. Moreover, genome-wide association studies have also identified numerous genomic loci that determine susceptibility to cardiovascular events [5]. Therefore, nutrition and genetics seem to interact in predisposing an individual to cardiovascular diseases [6]. The Special Issue "Nutrition, Genetics, and Cardiovascular Disease" of the *Journal of Cardiovascular Development and Disease* provided a platform for the presentation of recent advances in knowledge relating to nutrition, genetics and cardiovascular disease, from diverse scientific disciplines, and it included four original articles, one narrative review and one systematic review and meta-analysis.

The first original article investigated MT-CYB mutations in acute rheumatic fever and rheumatic heart diseases among Senegalese patients. The authors of this study found a narrow link between MT-CYB mutations and acute rheumatic fever and its complications, i.e., rheumatic heart diseases [7]. In the second original study, conducted in Uruguay on two separate cohorts (children, n = 682; adolescents, n = 340), the authors tested potential associations between anthropometric parameters (i.e., weight, height and body mass index (BMI)) in early life stages and the state of the cardiovascular system in early childhood at the beginning of adulthood [8]. The authors found that the current z-BMI showed the greatest capacity to explain variations in cardiovascular properties at 6 and 18 years. However, body size at birth showed no association with arterial properties at 6 or 18 years of age [8].

In the third original study, conducted in Saudi Arabia, the authors tested differences in dietary patterns (expressed in terms of adherence to the "Healthy Saudi" dietary guidelines) between two groups of males: CVD group (N = 40) and non-CVD group (N = 40) [9]. The authors found higher adherence scores for fruit, olive oil and non-alcoholic beer in the non-CVD patients [9]. The fourth original study, conducted on 460 healthy Lebanese adults from the general population, focused on detecting the association between the polymorphism rs2569190A > G in CD14 and CVD risk factors such as hypercholesterolemia and hypertension [10]. The authors found no significant association with hypertension. However, rs2569190G in CD14 was found to be associated with a higher risk of developing hypercholesterolemia among the Lebanese population [10].

On the other hand, the first systematic review that was conducted in Lebanon using the "Preferred Reporting Items for Systematic Reviews and Meta-Analyses" (PRISMA) guidelines in focused on clarifying whether hookah smoking is associated with a higher risk of obesity among the general population [11]. All the five included studies reported that hookah smoking increases the risk of obesity among all ages and in both genders, and this was confirmed by the meta-analysis [11]. Finally, in the narrative review of the renin angiotensin system (RAS) (known to be an endocrine system involved in blood-pressure regulation and body electrolyte balance) [12], the authors described the new components of RAS, their tissue-specific expression and their alterations under pathological conditions, which may facilitate development of more specific and personalized treatments [12].

In conclusion, the findings of the original articles and reviews of this Special Issue highlight certain nutritional and genetic features that seem to play an important role in CVDs.

Funding: This research received no external funding.

Conflicts of Interest: The authors declare no conflict of interest.

References

1. Stewart, J.; Manmathan, G.; Wilkinson, P. Primary prevention of cardiovascular disease: A review of contemporary guidance and literature. *JRSM Cardiovasc. Dis.* **2017**, *6*. [CrossRef] [PubMed]
2. McGavock, J.M.; Anderson, T.J.; Lewanczuk, R.Z. Sedentary Lifestyle and Antecedents of Cardiovascular Disease in Young Adults. *Am. J. Hypertens.* **2006**, *19*, 701–707. [CrossRef] [PubMed]
3. Ravera, A.; Carubelli, V.; Sciatti, E.; Bonadei, I.; Gorga, E.; Cani, D.S.; Vizzardi, E.; Metra, M.; Lombardi, C.M. Nutrition and Cardiovascular Disease: Finding the Perfect Recipe for Cardiovascular Health. *Nutrients* **2016**, *8*, 363. [CrossRef] [PubMed]
4. Poirier, P.; Giles, T.D.; Bray, G.A.; Hong, Y.; Stern, J.S.; Pi-Sunyer, F.X.; Eckel, R.H. Obesity and Cardiovascular Disease: Pathophysiology, Evaluation, and Effect of Weight Loss. *Circulation* **2006**, *113*, 898–918. [CrossRef] [PubMed]
5. Kathiresan, S.; Srivastava, D. Genetics of Human Cardiovascular Disease. *Cell* **2012**, *148*, 1242–1257. [CrossRef] [PubMed]
6. Said, M.A.; Van De Vegte, Y.J.; Zafar, M.; Van Der Ende, M.Y.; Raja, G.K.; Verweij, N.; Van Der Harst, P. Contributions of Interactions Between Lifestyle and Genetics on Coronary Artery Disease Risk. *Curr. Cardiol. Rep.* **2019**, *21*, 89. [CrossRef] [PubMed]
7. Wade, F.B.; Sall, M.P.; Mbaye, F.; Sembène, P.M. Mitochondrial DNA Mutations and Rheumatic Heart Diseases. *J. Cardiovasc. Dev. Dis.* **2019**, *6*, 36. [CrossRef] [PubMed]
8. Castro, J.M.; García-Espinosa, V.; Zinoveev, A.; Marin, M.; Severi, C.; Chiesa, P.; Bia, D.; Zócalo, Y. Arterial Structural and Functional Characteristics at End of Early Childhood and Beginning of Adulthood: Impact of Body Size Gain during Early, Intermediate, Late and Global Growth. *J. Cardiovasc. Dev. Dis.* **2019**, *6*, 33. [CrossRef] [PubMed]
9. Alkhaldy, A.A.; Alamri, R.S.; Magadmi, R.K.; Elshini, N.Y.; Hussein, R.A.E.H.; Alghalayini, K.W. Dietary Adherence of Saudi Males to the Saudi Dietary Guidelines and Its Relation to Cardiovascular Diseases: A Preliminary Cross-Sectional Study. *J. Cardiovasc. Dev. Dis.* **2019**, *6*, 17. [CrossRef] [PubMed]
10. Salami, A.; Costanian, C.; El Shamieh, S. rs2569190A>G in CD14 is Independently Associated with Hypercholesterolemia: A Brief Report. *J. Cardiovasc. Dev. Dis.* **2019**, *6*, 37. [CrossRef] [PubMed]
11. Baalbaki, R.; Itani, L.; El Kebbi, L.; Dehni, R.; Abbas, N.; Farsakouri, R.; Awad, D.; Tannir, H.; Kreidieh, D.; El Masri, D.; et al. Association Between Smoking Hookahs (Shishas) and Higher Risk of Obesity: A Systematic Review of Population-Based Studies. *J. Cardiovasc. Dev. Dis.* **2019**, *6*, 23. [CrossRef] [PubMed]
12. Nehme, A.; Zouein, F.A.; Zayeri, Z.D.; Zibara, K. An Update on the Tissue Renin Angiotensin System and Its Role in Physiology and Pathology. *J. Cardiovasc. Dev. Dis.* **2019**, *6*, 14. [CrossRef] [PubMed]

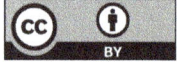

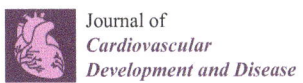

Journal of
Cardiovascular Development and Disease

Article

Mitochondrial DNA Mutations and Rheumatic Heart Diseases

Fatou Balla Wade *, Marie Parsine Sall, Fatimata Mbaye and Mbacké Sembene

Genetics and Population Management Team, Department of Animal Biology, Faculty of Sciences and Techniques, Cheikh Anta Diop University, Dakar 5005, Senegal; mparsine@yahoo.fr (M.P.S.);
fatimata.mbaye@ucad.edu.sn (F.M.); mbacke.sembene@ucad.edu.sn (M.S.)
* Correspondence: fatouballa.wade@ucad.edu.sn; Tel.: +221-78-117-51-77

Received: 2 September 2019; Accepted: 24 September 2019; Published: 11 October 2019

Abstract: Acute rheumatic fever (ARF) is an autoimmune disease affecting the heart-valve endocardium in its final stage. Although rare in developing countries, ARF persists in third-world countries, particularly Senegal, where rheumatic heart diseases (RHDs) are the most common pediatric cardiovascular pathology. This study aimed to investigate mutations in *MT-CYB* in ARF and RHD in Senegalese patients. *MT-CYB* was amplified from blood samples from ARF patients at the Clinical of Thoracic and Cardiovascular Surgery of Fann National University Hospital Centre, Dakar, Senegal (control group, healthy individuals) and sequenced. More than half of the *MT-CYB* mutations (58.23%) were heteroplasmic. Transitions (61.67%) were more frequent than transversions (38.33%), and non-synonymous substitutions represented 38.33% of mutations. Unoperated RHD patients harbored frequent *MT-CYB* polymorphisms (7.14 ± 14.70 mutations per sample) and accounted for 72.73% of mutations. Paradoxically, subjects undergoing valvular replacement harbored infrequent polymorphisms (1.39 ± 2.97 mutations per patient) and lacked 36 mutations present in unoperated subjects. A genetic differentiation was observed between these two populations, and the mutations in operated subjects were neutral, while those in unoperated subjects were under positive selection. These results indicate a narrow link (perhaps even causal) between *MT-CYB* mutations and ARF and its complications (i.e., RHDs) and that these mutations are largely deleterious.

Keywords: acute rheumatic fever; rheumatic heart diseases; *MT-CYB*; mutation; Senegal

1. Introduction

Acute rheumatic fever (ARF) is a major cause of cardiac disease and premature death in numerous regions worldwide [1]. ARF and rheumatic heart disease (RHD) have a high prevalence in developing countries in contrast with developed countries where these diseases have largely regressed [2]. ARF results in high morbidity and mortality rates worldwide and its incidence is the highest in Sub-Saharan Africa [3]. ARF incidence in developing countries exceeds 50 per 100,000 children [4]. In Senegal, RHD is the most prominent pediatric cardiovascular pathology [5].

Mutations in numerous genes, particularly those encoding immunity-related factors, are associated with ARF and RHD [6]. Genes encoding pattern recognition receptors belonging to the innate immune system, including ficolin [7], have been investigated. Genes encoding several cytokines including TNF-α or IL-6/-10 were reported to promote or aggravate ARF in studies in Mexico [8,9], Turkey [10], and Egypt [11].

On the other hand, it has been shown that the decrease in oxidative phosphorylation [12] Khatami mainly affects energy-intensive tissues, such as muscles, brain, heart, liver, and kidneys. This mechanism allows the production of ATP by the mitochondrial respiratory chain [13]. *MT-CYB* encodes the cytochrome b protein, which is the only subunit of the respiratory complex III (one of the five complexes of the respiratory chain), encoded by mitochondrial DNA, the others being of nuclear origin [13]. Cytochrome b plays a central role in the production of ATP [12] and as a catalytic subunit binding to the substrate of quinone and facilitating the transmission of electrons to cytochrome c [14]. Many mutations of *MT-CYB*, identified so far, are related to diseases such as stress intolerance, myopathies, cardiomyopathies, and neuropathies. These mutations generally show a deficit of enzymatic activity and a decrease in the number of certain subunits of complex III [13]. Mitochondrial dysfunction is characteristic of heart failure [15].

Thus far, no study on the mitochondrial genome has focused on ARF and RHD, and genetic investigations of these pathologies has not been carried out in Senegal. Hence, we hypothesized that mitochondrial *MT-CYB* mutations influence the occurrence and/or complications in ARF. This study aimed to investigate mutations in *MT-CYB* in ARF and RHD in Senegalese patients. The following were the objectives of our study: (1) To investigate *MT-CYB* polymorphisms in ARF; (2) to evaluate the genetic diversity of *MT-CYB* in ARF; (3) to determine the genetic structure of *MT-CYB* based on populations; (4) to identify the type of *MT-CYB* mutations in ARF.

2. Materials and Methods

2.1. Study Population

Patients with ARF undergoing follow-up examination at the Clinic of Thoracic and Cardiovascular Surgery of Fann National University Hospital Centre in Dakar, Senegal, were included herein. The study was approved by the ethics and research committee of Cheikh Anta Diop University (reference number: Protocol 0274/2018/CER/UCAD), and patients provided written informed consent prior to their participation in the study in accordance with the tenets of the Declaration of Helsinki. Some of these patients had undergone valvular replacement surgery, while others did not receive surgical intervention. Healthy individuals were recruited as controls.

Patients were divided into three groups: First group, healthy individuals (control group); second group, unoperated ARF patients; third group, operated ARF patients (n = 42 per group). In total, 126 blood samples obtained from each patient were stored in EDTA and labeled as Sg1, Sg2, etc.

2.2. Genetic Analysis

2.2.1. DNA Extraction and Amplification and Sequencing of MT-CYB

Genomic DNA was extracted using the DNase Blood Kit (Qiagen, South Korea) in accordance with the manufacturer's instructions. Polymerase chain reaction (PCR) was carried out to amplify *MT-CYB*, since it is reportedly involved in cardiovascular pathologies [12,15–19]. PCR amplification of *MT-CYB* was carried out at a reaction volume of 50 µL containing 2 µL of concentrated DNA and 48 µL of the PCR mix comprising 29.8 µL of MilliQ water, 5 µL of buffer, 1 µL of supplementary $MgCl_2$, 2 µL of dATP, dCTP, dGTP, and dTTP, 5 µL of H15915, 5 µL of L14723, and 0.2 µL of Tap polymerase. L14723 (5′-ACCAATGACATGAAAAATCATGGTT-3′) and H15915 (5′-TCTCCATTTCTGGTTTACAAGAC-3′) were the forward and reverse primers, respectively. The PCR program included the following conditions: 94 °C for 3 min; 40 cycles (94 °C for 45 s; 52 °C for 1 min; 72 °C 1 min for 30 s); 72 °C for 10 min. PCR products were purified and sequenced. Sequencing reactions were performed using an MJ Research PTC-225 Peltier thermocycler with the ABI PRISM kit and electrophoresed in an ABI 3730 XL sequencer.

2.2.2. Molecular Analyses

The chromatograms obtained after sequencing were submitted to the Mutation Surveyor software (https://softgenetics.com) version 5.0 to identify mutations and to determine their nature (homoplasmic or heteroplasmic) and their status (transition or transversion). Sequences of ARF with those of the controls. Mutation Surveyor assigned a score for each mutation, thus indicating the level of confidence regarding the accuracy of the cited base. Only those mutations with a score of ≥ 20 were retained (the probability that a cited base is false was 0.001; accuracy, 99%).

To determine the appropriate nucleotide position of our mutations in the mitochondrial genome, we performed BLASTn analysis (NCBI; https://ncbi.nlm.nih.gov/) with our raw control sequence. The position of each mutation and the corresponding amino acid was determined using BLASTx 2.8.0 [20], thus facilitating the identification of putative conserved domains [21].

To highlight the potential pathogenicity of non-synonymous mutations, we performed prediction analysis using three different software for transparency and reliability:

- POLYPHEN-2 [22], which yields the following putative results: Probably damaging ($p \leq 5\%$), potentially damaging ($5 < p \leq 10\%$), and benign ($p > 10\%$);
- SIFT [23], which assigns a score between zero and one. Amino acid substitutions are predicted to affect protein function when the score is ≤ 0.05 and to be tolerable when the score is >0.05;
- PROVEAN [24] wherein variants with a score of ≤ -2.5 are predicted as deleterious and those with a score of >-2.5 are considered neutral.

Non-synonymous *MT-CYB* mutations have been considered pathogenic if thus stipulated by at least two prediction software; if these mutations are not reported as neutral polymorphisms and if they are present in a conserved domain; heteroplasmy indicates high pathogenicity [25].

For further molecular analysis, we corrected and aligned sequences of ARF patients with those of the controls, using BioEdit version 7.1.9 [26] using the CLUSTALW algorithm [27]. Thereafter, we determined the following parameters underlying the genetic diversity of *MT-CYB* relative to each population, on the basis of which the groups were assessed and differentiated:

- The population size n corresponding to the number of individuals;
- The number of sites N that define the size of sequences;
- The variable sites, invariable sites, non-informative variables, and informative variables, the number of total mutations (Eta), thus elucidating *MT-CYB* polymorphisms in the study population;
- The number of haplotypes and the haplotype diversity (Hd), to analyze the distribution of individuals within a population;
- The nucleotide diversity (Pi) and the average number of nucleotide differences (k) that reflect genetic differences within a population.

These parameters were determined using DNAsp 5.10.01 [28]. Other parameters elucidating the genetic diversity are the following:

- The nucleotide frequencies: General and at each codon position;
- The nature of mutations (transitions and transversions);
- The rate of mutations (R);
- The rate of substitutions: Ks (synonymous) and Kns (non-synonymous).

These parameters were determined using Mega7 software version 7.0.26 [29], and the frequencies of amino acids was determined at the best reading frame (no stop codon).

For analysis using Mega7, it was necessary to determine the model describing the best pattern of substitution; hence, we used the following models:

- The HKY model [30] to control the population;
- The JC model [31] for unoperated ARF patients;
- The JC+G model [31] for operated ARF patients a gamma value of 0.06.

We used the Kimura 2-parameter model [32] to determine the rate of mutations because preferential models were unavailable for this analysis. The Nei-Gojobori modified model was used to estimate substitution rates.

Thereafter, we defined the parameters of genetic diversity among populations, thus highlighting *MT-CYB* polymorphisms in ARF patients. Using the DNAsp software, we estimated the following:

- The rate of nucleotide divergence representing the percentage of nucleotide-level differences in each generation;
- The nucleotide diversity between two populations;
- The average number of nucleotide-level differences at each site between pairwise sequences.

Further, we evaluated genetic differences and structural differences in *MT-CYB* in accordance with the study population. Using Mega7 version 7.0.26 [29], the genetic distances were determined, which facilitated the estimation of the rates of allele replacement among the compared entities, using the JC+G model (with G = 0.36), which was the most suitable model. To estimate genetic distances within populations, we used the K2 model, which is suitable for this analysis, while the JC+G model was not. Furthermore, we estimated the genetic distance between the control population and ARF patients (operated and unoperated). For all analyses of genetic distances, the bootstrap method was used with 1000 replicates and all reading frames were accounted for. Using Arlequin version 3.1 [33], we estimated the genetic differentiation factor (Fst) between populations and performed analysis of molecular variance (AMOVA) to determine the origin of the variants. These analyses were performed considering polymorphic loci only and with 1023 permutations.

The Z-test for selection was performed using Mega7 in accordance with three different alternative hypotheses, the null hypothesis being that H0: dN = dS. We then assessed the neutral selection (H_1: dN ≠ dS), the positive selection (dN > dS), and the negative selection (dN < dS). We used the Nei-Gojobori modified model [34], which differs from the original method of Nei-Gojobori in that transitional and transversional substitutions were no longer considered to occur at the same frequency. Thus, we calculated the ratio of transitions/transversions with the following formula [30]:

$$\kappa = \frac{(\pi t \pi c + \pi a \pi g)}{\pi y \pi r} \alpha / \beta \tag{1}$$

where πa, πc, πg, and πt are the nucleotide frequencies (of a, c, g, and t, respectively) estimated by their proportions in all sequences: $\pi y = \pi t + \pi c$ and $\pi r = \pi a + \pi g$; α and β are the number of transitions and transversions, respectively, observed by considering all sequences in a pairwise manner.

2.3. Statistical Analyses

Data normality was assessed using XLSTAT 2018.3.50896 with the Shapiro-Wilk test with a rate of significance level set to 5%. We then performed the Fisher test (for non-normally distributed data) to establish an association between mutations and the state of the disease, always at a threshold of 5%. Mean and standard deviation values for mutations were determined using MS Excel 2010 and compared using R commander (Rcmdr) implemented in RGui version 3.3.4 to assess differences between operated and unoperated ARF patients.

Average amino acid frequencies of the controls and unoperated AFR patients and between the controls and operated ARF patients were compared using the chi-square test in Rstudio version 1.1.447. Since chi-square analysis is only feasible when the number of groups is <5, we used complementary values (100-effective).

3. Results

3.1. Evaluation of MT-CYB Polymorphisms

3.1.1. Analysis of MT-CYB Mutations

BLASTn analysis revealed 97% identity with *MT-CYB* and 5 gaps. BLASTx analysis revealed 98% identity (without gaps) with the cytochrome b (mitochondrion) [*Homo sapiens*] [35] and [*Homo sapiens subsp. 'Denisova'*] [36] and 97% identity (without gaps) with cytochrome b (mitochondrion) [*Homo heidelbergensis*] [37] and [*Homo sapiens neanderthalensis*] [38].

Alignment of the chromatograms of ARF patients (operated and unoperated) with those of the controls (Sg97) revealed 165-point mutations with a score of ≥20 or 60 different variants, in the overall study population. Among them, 41.67% corresponded with homoplasmic mutations and 58.23% corresponded with heteroplasmic mutations. Transitions largely surpassed the transversions (respectively 61.67% and 38.33%). Most mutations were present in unoperated ARF patients (72.73%) wherein 7.14 ± 14.70 mutations on average were harbored per individual. Indeed, seven mutations were present at high frequencies in ARF patients (G15849A, T15824C, A15784G, A15362T, A15323C, G15314C, and A15308T). Synonymous (A15362T and A15323C) and missense (G15314C and A15308T) mutations were exclusively present in unoperated ARF patients at frequencies of 67.86%, 67.86%, 42.86%, and 57.14%, respectively. The Fisher test revealed significant results for these mutations, thus indicating their association with ARF. Overall, 36 mutations were absent in the operated ARF patients. Thus, operated ARF patients harbored 1.39 ± 2.97 mutations on average. Differences in the average mutation frequencies were significant (p = 0.031). The frequency for synonymous mutations was 38.33% among the ARF patients. Among these amino acid substitutions, nine were pathogenic according to the predictions of Polyphen-2, SIFT, and PROVEAN. All the pathogenic mutations were absent in the operated patients, except for the missense substitutions K287P and N286P, present in all positions of their corresponding codons and present in only one subject (Sg56). Most mutated sites were detected through MITOMAP (https://www.mitomap.org/MITOMAP); however, the corresponding bases differed from the those in the present sequences (Table 1).

3.1.2. Variability of Amino Acids

Transcription was carried out based on the second reading frame. Gly and Leu were the most frequent amino acids in the protein. Asn and His were absent in the ARF patients and the controls. Pro and Thr were absent in the controls but present at low frequencies in the ARF patients. However, none of the P-values is significant (Table 2).

3.1.3. Determination of Genetic Diversity of MT-CYB

The analysis of the genetic diversity of the study population is summarized in Table 3. In the study population, 12, 28, and 54 individuals belonged to the control, unoperated, and operated groups, respectively. The sizes of the sequences were the same for each individual (492 bp). The unoperated group differed from the other two groups and displayed the highest *MT-CYB* polymorphism frequency. The nucleotide frequencies were similar in all groups. Cytosine was the least represented base with a minimal frequency at the third codon position in contrast with thymine and guanine, which were more frequent at this position. Adenine occurred mostly at the first codon position. In position 1, no transversions occurred, and all mutations were transitions (conservation of the mutated base); hence, the mutation rate (R) tended towards infinity.

Table 1. Characteristics of MT-CYB mutations.

Mutations	Rate	p. rCRS	Proportions of Mutations			Status	Nature	P. AA	CD	PolyPhen-2 Prediction	Sift Prediction	Provean Prediction	Conclusion	References
			S %	NO %	O %									
T69C	91	15851	1.22	3.57	0.00	Homo	T	I369V	Yes	Benign 0	TOL	Neutral	N.P	+ (A > C) (1)
G71A	142	15849	9.76	10.71	9.26 *	Homo	T	T368I	Yes	Benign 0	TOL	Neutral	N.P	+ (C > T)
G81GC	20	15839	1.22	3.57	0.00	Hetero	T	L365L	Yes					+ (C > T)
A89AT	22	15831	1.22	3.57	0.00	Hetero	T	I362I	Yes					
T94TA	83	15826	1.22	3.57	0.00	Hetero	T	T360T	Yes					
T96C	101	15824	15.85	21.43	12.96 *	Homo	T	T360A	Yes	Benign 0	TOL	Neutral	N.P	+ (A > G)
T121C	119	15799	1.22	0.00 *	1.85	Homo	T	Q352Q	Yes					+ (A > G)
G130A	103	15790	2.44	0.00	3.70 *	Homo	T	T348T	Yes					+ (C > T)
A133AC	21	15787	1.22	0.00 *	1.85	Hetero	T	F347F	Yes					+ (C > T)
A136G	86	15784	14.63	10.71 *	16.67 *	Homo	T	P346P	Yes					+ (C > T) (3)
A136AG	45	15784	1.22	0.00 *	1.85	Hetero	T	P346P	Yes					+ (C > T) (3)
A141AT	25	15779	1.22	3.57	0.00	Hetero	T	Y345Y	Yes					+ (T > C)
C143G	150	15777	1.22	3.57	0.00	Homo	T	S344T	Yes	p.D	AFP	Neutral	P	+ (G > C)
T162C	146	15758	2.44	0.00	3.70 *	Homo	T	I338V	Yes	Benign	AFP	Neutral	N.P	+ (A > G) (1)
G171GC	25	15749	3.66	3.57	3.70	Hetero	T	L335L	Yes					+ (C > T)
G177GC	23	15743	1.22	3.57	0.00	Hetero	t	L333L	Yes					+ (C > T)
C186T	119	15734	1.22	3.57	0.00	Homo	T	A330T	Yes	Benign	AFP	Neutral	N.P	+ (G > A)
G187GC	28	15733	1.22	0.00 *	1.85	Hetero	t	A330A	Yes					+ (C > A)
A250G	99	15670	2.44	7.14	0.00 *	Homo	T	H308H	Yes					+ (T > C)
A254AT	36	15666	1.22	0.00 *	1.85	Hetero	t	L307L	Yes					

Table 1. *Cont.*

Mutations	Rate	p. rCRS	Proportions of Mutations			Status	Nature	p. AA	CD	PolyPhen-2 Prediction	Sift Prediction	Provean Prediction	Conclusion	References
			S %	NO %	O %									
G256A	151	15664	1.22	3.57	0.00	Homo	T	I306I	Yes					+ (C > A)
A257AG	40	15663	1.22	3.57	0.00	Hetero	T	I306I	Yes					+ (T > C)
T267TG	24	15653	1.22	0.00 *	1.85	Hetero	t	M303M	Yes					+ (A > G)
G279GA	40	15641	2.44	7.14	0.00 *	Hetero	T	L299F	Yes	P:D	AFP	Neutral	P	+ (C > T)
A281AG	**44**	**15639**	**1.22**	**3.57**	**0.00**	**Hetero**	**T**	**I298T**	**Yes**	**P:D**	**AFP**	**Del**	**P**	**+ (T > C)**
A287AC	32	15633	1.22	0.00 *	1.85	Hetero	T	L296L	Yes					+ (C > T)
G288GA	24	15632	1.22	3.57	0.00	Hetero	T	L296L	Yes					+ (T > C)
A291AG	22	15629	1.22	3.57	0.00	Hetero	T	L295L	Yes					+ (C > T)
G294A	41	15626	1.22	0.00 *	1.85	Homo	T	L294L	Yes					+ (C > T)
G304C	23	15616	1.22	0.00 *	1.85	Homo	T	G290G	Yes					+ (A > G)
T307C	48	15613	1.22	0.00 *	1.85	Homo	T	G289G	Yes					(1)(2)(3)
T313C	70	15607	1.22	0.00 *	1.85	Homo	T	K287P	Yes	P:D	AFP	Del	P	
T314TC	50	15606	1.22	0.00 *	1.85	Hetero	T	K287P	Yes	P:D	AFP	Del	P	
T315TC	50	15605	1.22	0.00 *	1.85	Hetero	T	K287P	Yes	P:D	AFP	Del	P	
G316GC	44	15604	1.22	0.00 *	1.85	Hetero	T	N286P	Yes	P:D	TOL	Del	P	+ (C > T)
T317TC	45	15603	1.22	0.00 *	1.85	Hetero	T	N286P	Yes	P:D	TOL	Del	P	+ (A > G)
T318TC	38	15602	1.22	0.00 *	1.85	Hetero	T	N286P	Yes	P:D	TOL	Del	P	
A319G	128	15601	1.22	3.57	0.00	Homo	T	P285P	Yes					+ (T > C)
A319AG	58	15601	2.44	7.14	0.00 *	Hetero	T	P285P	Yes					
G320GC	22	15600	1.22	0.00 *	1.85	Hetero	T	P285P	Yes					

Table 1. *Cont.*

Mutations	Rate	p. rCRS	Proportions of Mutations			Status	Nature	p. AA	CD	PolyPhen-2 Prediction	Sift Prediction	Provean Prediction	Conclusion	References
			S %	NO %	O %									
G321GC	106	15599	1.22	0.00 *	1.85	Hetero	T	P285P	Yes					
A323AG	24	15597	1.22	3.57	0.00	Hetero	T	V284V	Yes					
A342G	23	15578	1.22	3.57	0.00	Hetero	T	Y278Y	Yes					
G343GC	35	15577	1.22	3.57	0.00	Hetero	T	A277A	Yes					
A390AG	73	15530	1.22	3.57	0.00	Hetero	T	L262L	Yes					+ (T > C) (1)
C454CT	31	15466	2.44	7.14	0.00 *	Hetero	T	M240M	Yes					+ (G > A)
G460GA	44	15460	1.22	3.57	0.00	Hetero	T	S238L	Yes	Benign	TOL	Neutral	N.P	+ (C > T)
A466AG	24	15454	2.44	7.14	0.00 *	Hetero	T	L236L	Yes					+ (T > C)
G487GA	24	15433	1.22	3.57	0.00	Hetero	T	A229A	Yes					+ (C > T)
G534C	**149**	**15386**	**1.22**	**3.57**	**0.00**	**Homo**	**T**	**H214D**	**Yes**	**Benign**	**TOL**	**Neutral**	**N.P**	**+ (C > A)**
G539A	148	15381	1.22	3.57	0.00	Homo	T	T212I	Yes	Benign	TOL	Neutral	N.P	+ (C > T)
A558T	80	15362	23.17	67.86 *	0.00 *	Homo	T	Y206Y	Yes					
A597C	128	15323	23.17	67.86 *	0.00 *	Homo	T	S193S	No					+ (G > A)
G606C	32	15314	14.63	42.86 *	0.00 *	Homo	T	T190A	No					+ (G > A)
T609C	49	15311	3.66	10.71	0.00 *	Homo	T	L189V	No	Benign	TOL	-	N.P	+ (A > G)
A610AC	21	15310	1.22	3.57	0.00	Hetero	T	F188I	No					+ (T > C)
A610GA	66	15310	1.22	3.57	0.00	Homo	T	F188I	No					+ (T > C)
A612T	42	15308	19.51	57.14 *	0.00 *	Homo	T	F188I	No					+ (A > G)
G616GA	43	15304	1.22	3.57	0.00	Hetero	T	P186P	No					+ (C > T)
T619C	45	15301	3.66	10.71	0.00 *	Homo	T	I185L	No					+ (G > A) (3)

Rate: Mutation rates determined via Mutation Surveyor; **p. rCRS**: Position according to the Cambridge reference sequence; **S**: ARF patients; **NO**: Unoperated; **O**: Operated; **p.AA**: Amino acid position according to the protein reference sequence (UniProt accession number: P00156); **CD**: Conserved domain [MT-CYB (52-570) preserved in mammals; Cytochrom_B_C (97-399) preserved in cellular organisms; QcrB (97-564) preserved in cellular organisms; cytochrome_b_C (115-555) containing the redox sites of quinol and the polypeptide binding site, preserved in cellular organisms; MT-CYB6/f-IV (301-435) preserved in cellular organisms]; **Homo**: Homoplasmic mutation; **Hetero**: Heteroplasmic mutation; **T**: Transition; **t**: Transversion; **(1)**: [14] (A > G); **(2)**: [39] (T > C); **(3)**: [16] (A > G); **NP**: Not pathogenic; **P**: Pathogenic; **P.D**: Probably damaging; **p.D**: Potentially damaging; **TOL**: Tolerable; **Del**: Deleterious; ***: Significant Fisher; +: Listed in MITOMAP, the letters in parentheses represent the referenced substitutions.

Table 2. Frequencies of amino acids according to populations.

Amino Acids	Controls	Operated	Non-Operated	P-Value C vs. O	P-Value C vs. NOP	P-Value O vs. NOP
Ala	0.67	0.68	0.69	0.999	0.999	0.999
Cys	4.72	4.68	4.74	0.997	0.999	0.996
Asp	0.00	0.00	0.00	1	1	1
Glu	3.89	3.96	3.96	0.996	0.997	0.999
Phe	2.67	2.70	2.69	0.998	0.999	0.999
Gly	21.40	21.20	21.06	0.987	0.978	0.999
His	0.00	0.00	0.00	1	1	1
Ile	2.67	2.68	2.67	0.999	1	0.992
Lys	2.00	1.93	2.07	0.996	0.996	0.998
Leu	20.68	20.73	20.71	0.997	0.998	1
Met	6.00	6.01	6.00	0.999	0.999	1
Asn	2.67	2.67	2.67	1	1	1
Pro	0.00	0.04	0.07	0.998	0.996	0.998
Gln	1.33	1.34	1.43	1	0.995	0.995
Arg	7.34	7.52	7.46	0.989	0.993	0.996
Ser	3.34	3.36	3.34	0.998	1	0.998
Thr	0.00	0.01	0.05	0.999	0.997	0.999
Val	10.01	9.91	9.89	0.994	0.993	0.999
Trp	8.62	8.57	8.58	0.997	0.998	0.999
Tyr	2.00	2.00	1.93	1	0.996	0.996

C: Controls, O: Operated, NOP: Unoperated.

Table 3. Parameters for genetic diversity of the study population.

Parameters		Controls				Unoperated				Operated		
Size of population n		12				28				54		
Number of sites N		492				492				492		
Non-variables sites		485				441				450		
Variables sites		7				51				42		
Non-informative variables sites		5				43				25		
Informative variables sites		2				8				17		
Number of total mutations Eta		7				52				52		
Number of haplotypes		7				17				29		
Haplotypic diversity hd		0.833 ± 0.100				0.923 ± 0.037				0.883 ± 0.039		
Nucleotide diversity Pi		0.00314 ± 0.00071				0.00996 ± 0.00336				0.00645 ± 0.00129		
The average number of nucleotide differences k		1.545				4.902				3.173		
Nucleotide frequencies		T	C	A	G	T	C	A	G	T	C	A	G
General		29.5	9.3	25.2	36.0	29.4	9.5	25.3	35.8	29.5	9.5	25.2	35.9
Position 1		21	9.8	27.4	21	9.7	42.1	27.4	21	9.8	42.0	27.3	42.1
Position 2		29	17.1	20.8	32.9	29	17.4	20.9	32.5	29	17.3	20.8	32.6
Position 3		38	1.2	12.7	47.7	38	1.4	12.8	47.5	38	1.3	12.7	47.6
Nature of mutations	Transitions	100				46.92				34.91		
	Transversions	0				53.08				65.09		
Rate of mutations R		∞				0.88				0.54		
Rate of synonymous substitutions Ks		0.002 ± 0.001				0.011 ± 0.003				0.006 ± 0.003		
Rate of non-synonymous substitutions Kns		0.003 ± 0.002				0.007 ± 0.002				0.005 ± 0.002		

3.1.4. Evaluation of the Differentiation and Genetic Structuring of MT-CYB in Accordance with the Study Population

The genetic distance was the largest among unoperated ARF patients (0.011 ± 0.002) and the lowest in the controls (0.003 ± 0.001). Genetic distances were greater between unoperated and operated

ARF patients (0.009 ± 0.001) than between the controls and operated ARF patients (0.005 ± 0.001) (Table 4).

Analysis of the genetic differentiation factor (Fst) revealed no genetic differentiation of *MT-CYB* between the controls and patients (p = 0.58559). However, a genetic differentiation of *MT-CYB* between operated and unoperated subjects was observed (p = 0.01466) (Table 5). Nevertheless, AMOVA (Table 6) revealed that more than 98% of genetic variability between unoperated and operated ARF patients is of an intra-population origin.

Table 4. Genetic distances within and among groups.

	Controls	**Non-Operated**	**Operated**
Controls	0.003 ± 0.001		
Non-operated	0.007 ± 0.001	**0.011 ± 0.002**	
Operated	0.005 ± 0.001	0.009 ± 0.001	0.007 ± 0.001

In boldface: The highest genetic distances.

Table 5. Genetic differentiation factor.

	Controls	**Unoperated**	**Operated**
Controls		*0.87195*	*0.38416*
Unoperated	0		***0.01466***
Operated	0.00128	0.01419	

In italics, the p-values and in bold the significant p-value.

Table 6. Analysis of molecular variance.

Source of Variation	**Percentage Variation**
Inter-populations	1.41855
Intra-population	98.58145

3.1.5. Evolution of MT-CYB Mutations

As shown in Table 7, the results of the Z selection test among groups were recorded. The non-significant p-values (0.965, 0.483, and 1.000) among operated ARF patients indicate that their mutations follow a neutral evolution. However, among unoperated ARF patients, the p-value, highly significant under the neutrality hypothesis (0.015), highly significant under the hypothesis of positive selection, and not significant under the hypothesis of negative selection, shows that *MT-CYB* mutations in the unoperated patients are under positive selection.

Table 7. Results of the Z selection test (p-values).

	Neutrality	**Positive Selection**	**Negative Selection**
Operated	0.965	0.483	1.000
Non-operated	**0.015**	**0.008**	1.000

In boldface: Significant p-values.

4. Discussion

This study attempted to identify *MT-CYB* mutations in Senegalese ARF patients. Since cardiac tissues were not available for molecular analysis, mutations in this region were assessed in peripheral blood. The present results show a high rate of *MT-CYB* polymorphisms in unoperated subjects (72.73% of mutations). Unoperated ARF patients developed a cardiopathy following ARF; however, since they did not undergo valvular replacement, the disease was seemingly induced in them, and *MT-CYB* mutations were detected in the cells involved in the autoimmune response in blood, similar to T and B lymphocytes, and macrophages, since self-reactive T cells migrate from peripheral blood to the heart and proliferate in the valves in response to stimulation by specific cytokines [6].

Two synonymous substitutions (Y206Y and S193S) associated with ARF (according to the Fisher test) were observed at high frequencies (67.86%) and exclusively in the operated subjects. Despite the absence of amino acid substitutions, the corresponding positions (A15362T and A15323C) may serve as potential molecular markers if consistently present in individuals with ARF. Non-synonymous substitutions T190A, F188I, and I185L, frequent in the unoperated group, are also associated with the pathology. These sites were polymorphic in comparison with the control but monomorphic in comparison with the Caucasian reference sequence. These mutations were detected on MITOMAP but matched with different substitutions. The mutation T15301C (I185L) is associated with idiopathic dilated cardiomyopathy [14] as being a synonymous substitution Leu-Leu. Three missense mutations (S344T, L299F, and I298T), predicted to be pathogenic, have been reported in unoperated patients 2 and 1. The substitution of an aliphatic Leu with an aromatic Phe and that of nonpolar Ile with a polar Thr affected protein structure and function. The substitution of Ser with Thr could have been inconsequential, since they are both thiolated/hydroxylated and polar amino acids and the mutation is homoplasmic (the predictions of this mutation are not formal; thus, mutation may be benign). However, these mutations are in a conserved domain, playing a crucial role in cytochrome b function and thus in the activity of complex III. The C-terminal domain contains the binding sites for ubiquinone/ubiquinol [40,41] and is responsible for proton translocation outside the mitochondrial membrane [42]. Furthermore, the L299F mutation has been reported in breast cancer; however, it was a substitution from cytosine to thymine (according to the reference sequence) at position 15641, whereas the mutation detected herein corresponds to the heteroplasmic substitution of guanine by adenine (according to our control sequence). Both mutations were transitions occurring in the same position. Several mutations were present in both unoperated and operated patients, including G15849A and T15824C synonymous substitutions and the A15784G sense mutation. G15849A and T15824C corresponding to substitutions T368I and T360A have been predicted to be non-pathogenic, although they are polar Thr substitutions by non-polar Ile and Ala. These point mutations occur in a conserved domain in mammals, but are outside the C-terminal domain, thus probably accounting for their benign state. T15824C is present in breast cancer as A15824G, and A15784G has been reported in patients with dilated idiopathic cardiomyopathy [16]. Most (60%) of the mutations were absent in operated patients. Mutations present only in the latter were either synonymous or non-pathogenic, except for those present in one patient (Sg56). More than half of the *MT-CYB* mutations were heteroplasmic (58.23%), probably because polymorphonuclear mitochondrial genomes do not contain *MT-CYB* mutations leading to a mixture of wildtype and mutated genomes or heteroplasmy in immune cells. Cells were not isolated for DNA extraction; either of the hypotheses cannot be considered accurate. However, the current speculation that heteroplasmic mutations are more likely to occur in pathogenic mutations rather than in normal polymorphisms [16] is consistent with the present pathogenic mutations.

Amino acid frequencies did not differ significantly upon pairwise group comparisons. However, Pro and Thr were absent in the controls but present in ARF patients at low frequencies, indeed because of the presence of missense mutations.

Differences in the degree of *MT-CYB* polymorphisms between operated and unoperated patients suggest that valvular replacement suppressed gene mutations. This is corroborated by the results of the genetic diversity of the study population, which facilitated the characterization and analysis of differences between unoperated ARF patients and the other two groups in the study population. Similarly, group comparisons in the study population revealed the genetic proximity of operated subjects and the controls (Pi, k, and the genetic distances were low) and those genetic differences between the operated and unoperated patients. These results may have been obtained because surgery eliminates diseased valvular cells and simultaneously the source of the pathology. The proteins of valvular cells similar to those of *Streptococcus pyogenes* [43] are the targets of immune cells. Eradication of the source of the pathology would lead to a correction between the mechanism underlying autoimmunity, and the cells involved in the defense against *Streptococcus* of Group A and autoimmunity would become functional again in the next generation. Selection analyses have indicated that mutations in the operated subjects follow a neutral evolution, while those present in the unoperated patients are under positive selection. These results are concurrent with previous findings; non-synonymous *MT-CYB* mutations tend to consistently occur in unoperated patients. These variants have a deleterious effect on the protein, and an increase in their frequency would further cause protein damage and simultaneously aggravate the disease. Since these mutations generally do not occur in operated patients and those persisting after valvular replacement are neutral (neither beneficial nor deleterious), the involvement of *MT-CYB* mutations in ARF complications can be considered (RHD).

5. Conclusions

This study used a population genetics approach to investigate the association of *MT-CYB* mutations with ARF and RHD in Senegalese patients. The present results confirmed our initial hypothesis. Indeed, sixty polymorphic variants of *MT-CYB* were identified herein. Some of these mutations were neutral, while other mutations were pathogenic, as revealed through their effects on cytochrome b structure and function. Furthermore, the absence of more than half of these mutations in patients with valvular replacement and genetic differentiation between the latter and unoperated patients indicates *MT-CYB* polymorphisms, which are closely associated with ARF and RHD. These mutations cause or result from abnormal activation of immune cells against autoantigens. A study combining both immune assessment with a genetics approach would be interesting to clarify why only some individuals infected with group A streptococcus develop an inadequate immune response leading to ARF. A subsequent analysis of the protein would also provide useful insights into the role of cytochrome b in ARF and RHD. In addition, DNA extraction in the same patient before and after surgery could validate our results.

Author Contributions: Conceptualization, F.B.W. and F.M.; Data curation, F.B.W.; Formal analysis, F.B.W.; Investigation, F.B.W. and M.P.S.; Methodology, F.B.W.; Project administration, F.M.; Resources, M.S.; Software, F.B.W.; Supervision, F.M. and M.S.; Validation, F.M. and M.S.; Visualization, F.B.W. and F.M.; Writing—original draft, F.B.W.; Writing—review and editing, F.M.

Funding: This research received no external funding.

Conflicts of Interest: The authors declare no conflict of interest.

References

1. Bryant, P.A.; Robins-Browne, R.; Carapetis, J.R.; Curtis, N. Some of the People, Some of the Time: Susceptibility to Acute Rheumatic Fever. *Circulation* **2009**, *119*, 742–753. [CrossRef] [PubMed]
2. Templeton, C.G.; Cooper, A.R.; Human, D.G.; Rahman, P. Rhumatisme articulaire aigu. *Le Programme Canadien de Surveillance Pédiatrique*, Unpublished. 2007; 4p.
3. Venter, M.; Van der Westhuizen, F.H.; Elson, J.L. The aetiology of cardiovascular disease: A role for mitochondrial DNA? *Cardiovasc. J. Afr.* **2017**, *29*, 122–132. [CrossRef] [PubMed]
4. Carapetis, J.R.; Steer, A.; Mulholland, E.; Weber, M. The global burden of group A streptococcal disease. *Lancet Infect. Dis.* **2005**, *5*, 685–694. [CrossRef]
5. Fall, A.L.; Ndiaye, O.; Lavou, I.; Sow, H.D. La cardiopathie rhumatismale à l'Hôpital d'Enfants Albert Royer de Dakar: À propos de 76 cas. In Proceedings of the Conférence IVème Congrès de l'Association des Pédiatres d'Afrique Noire Francophone (APANF) et IIème Congrès de la Société Sénégalaise de Pédiatrie (SOSEPED), Dakar, Senegal, November 2007. Résumé.
6. Guilherme, L.; Köhler, K.F.; Postol, E.; Kalil, J. Genes, autoimmunity and pathogenesis of rheumatic heart disease. *Ann. Paediatr. Cardiol.* **2011**, *4*, 13–21. [CrossRef] [PubMed]

7. Messias-Reason, I.J.; Schafranski, M.D.; Kremsner, P.G.; Kun, J.F. Ficolin 2 (FCN2) functional polymorphisms and the risk of rheumatic fever and rheumatic heart disease. *Clin. Exp. Immunol.* **2009**, *157*, 395–399. [CrossRef] [PubMed]

8. Hernández-Pacheco, G.; Flores-Domínguez, C.; Rodríguez-Pérez, J.M.; Pérez-Hernández, N.; Fragoso, J.M.; Saul, A.; Vargas-Alarcón, G. Tumour necrosis factor-alpha promoter polymorphisms in Mexican patients with rheumatic heart disease. *J. Autoimmun.* **2003**, *21*, 59–63. [CrossRef]

9. Sallakci, N.; Akcurin, G.; Köksoy, S.; Kardelen, F.; Uguz, A.; Coskun, M.; Yegin, O. TNF-alpha G-308A polymorphism is associated with rheumatic fever and correlates with increased TNF-alpha production. *J. Autoimmun.* **2005**, *25*, 150–154. [CrossRef]

10. Yeğin, O.; Coşkun, M.; Ertuğ, H. Cytokines in acute rheumatic fever. *Eur. J. Paediatr.* **1997**, *156*, 25–29. [CrossRef]

11. Settin, A.; Abdel-Hady, H.; El-Baz, R.; Saber, I. Gene polymorphisms of TNF-alpha^{-308}, IL-10^{-108}, IL-6^{-174}, and IL-1Ra^{VNTR} related to susceptibility and severity of rheumatic heart disease. *Paediatr. Cardiol.* **2007**, *28*, 363–371. [CrossRef]

12. Marin-Garcia, J.; Ananthakrishnan, R.; Gonzalvo, A.; Goldenthal, M.J. Novel mutations in mitochondrial cytochrome b in fatal post-partum cardiomyopathy. *J. Inherit. Metab. Dis.* **1995**, *18*, 77–78. [CrossRef]

13. Ekiert, R.; Borek, A.; Kuleta, P.; Czernek, J.; Osyczka, A. Mitochondrial disease-related mutations at the cytochrome b-iron–sulfur protein (ISP) interface: Molecular effects on the large-scale motion of ISP and superoxide generation studied in Rhodobacter capsulatus cytochrome bc1. *Biochim. Biophys. Acta* **2016**, *1857*, 1102–1110. [CrossRef] [PubMed]

14. Andreu, A.L.; Bruno, C.; Hadjigeorgiou, G.M.; Shanske, S.; DiMauro, S. Polymorphic Variants in the Human Mitochondrial Cytochrome b Gene. *Mol. Genet. Metab.* **1999**, *67*, 49–52. [CrossRef]

15. Hagen, C.H.; Aidt, F.H.; Havndrup, O.; Hedley, P.L.; Jespersgaard, C.; Jensen, M.; Christiansen, M. MT-CYB mutations in hypertrophic cardiomyopathy. *Mol. Genet. Genom. Med.* **2013**, *1*, 54–65. [CrossRef] [PubMed]

16. Marin-Garcia, J.; Goldenthal, M.J.; Ananthakrishnan, R.; Pierpont, M.E. The Complete Sequence of mtDNA Genes in Idiopathic Dilated Cardiomyopathy Shows Novel Missense and tRNA Mutations. *J. Card. Fail.* **2000**, *6*, 321–329. [CrossRef] [PubMed]

17. Andreu, A.L.; Checcarelli, N.; Iwata, S.; Shanske, S.; Dimauro, S. Missense Mutation in the Mitochondrial Cytochrome b Gene in a Revisited Case with Histiocytoid Cardiomyopathy. *Pediatr. Res.* **2000**, *48*, 311–314. [CrossRef] [PubMed]

18. Wang, J.; Lin, F.; Guo, L.; Xiong, X.; Fan, X. Cardiovascular Disease, Mitochondria, and Traditional Chinese Medicine. *Evidence-Based Complement. Med.* **2015**, *2015*, 1–7. [CrossRef]

19. Khatami, M.; Heidari, M.M.; Karimian, N.; Hadadzadeh, M. Mitochondrial Mutations in tRNAGlu and Cytochrome b Genes Associated with Iranian Congenial Heart Disease. *Int. Cardiovasc. Res. J.* **2016**, *10*, 193–198.

20. Altschul, S.F.; Madden, T.L.; Schäffer, A.A.; Zhang, J.; Zhang, Z.; Miller, W.; Lipman, D.J. Gapped BLAST and PSI-BLAST: A new generation of protein database search programs. *Nucleic Acids Res.* **1997**, *25*, 3389–3402. [CrossRef]

21. Geer, L.Y.; Domrachev, M.; Lipman, D.J.; Bryant, S.H. CDART: Protein homology by domain architecture. *Genome Res.* **2002**, *12*, 1619–1623. [CrossRef]

22. Adzhubei, I.; Jordan, D.; Sunyaev, S. Predicting functional effect of human missense mutations using PolyPhen-2. *Curr. Protoc. Hum. Genet.* **2013**, *7*, 1–52. [CrossRef]

23. Pauline, C.N.; Steven, H. Predicting Deleterious Amino Acid Substitutions. *Genome Res.* **2001**, *11*, 863–874.

24. Choi, Y.; Sims, G.E.; Murphy, S.; Miller, J.R.; Chan, A.P. Predicting the Functional Effect of Amino Acid Substitutions and Indels. *PLoS ONE* **2012**, *7*, 1–13. [CrossRef] [PubMed]

25. Chinnery, P.F.; Howell, N.; Andrews, R.M.; Turnbull, D.M. Mitochondrial DNA analysis: Polymorphisms and pathogenicity. *J. Med. Genet.* **1999**, *36*, 505–510. [CrossRef] [PubMed]

26. Hall, T.A. BioEdit: A user-friendly biological sequence alignment editor and analysis program for Windows 95/98/NT. *Nucleic Acids Symp. Ser.* **1999**, *41*, 95–98.

27. Thompson, J.D.; Higgins, D.G.; Gibson, T.J. CLUSTAL W: Improving the sensitivity of progressive multiple sequence alignment through sequence weighting, position-specific gap penalties and weight matrix choice. *Nucleic Acids Res.* **1994**, *22*, 4673–4680. [CrossRef] [PubMed]

28. Librado, P.; Rozas, J. DnaSP v5: A software for comprehensive analysis of DNA polymorphism data. *Bioinformatics* **2009**, *25*, 1451–1452. [CrossRef] [PubMed]

29. Kumar, S.; Stecher, G.; Tamura, K. MEGA7: Molecular Evolutionary Genetics Analysis version 7.0 for bigger datasets. *Mol. Biol. Evol.* **2016**, *33*, 1870–1874. [CrossRef] [PubMed]

30. Hasegawa, M.; Kishino, H.; Yano, T. Dating the human-ape split by a molecular clock of mitochondrial DNA. *J. Mol. Evol.* **1985**, *22*, 160–174. [CrossRef]

31. Jukes, T.; Cantor, C. Evolution of protein molecules. In *Mammalian Protein Metabolism*; Munro, H.N., Ed.; Academic Press: New York, NY, USA, 1969; p. 21.

32. Kimura, M. A simple method for estimating evolutionary rate of base substitutions through comparative studies of nucleotide sequences. *J. Mol. Evolut.* **1980**, *16*, 111–120. [CrossRef]

33. Excoffier, L. *Computational and Molecular Population Genetics Lab CMPG*; Zoological Institute, University of Berne: Bern, Switzerland, 2006.

34. Nei, M.; Gojobori, T. Simple methods for estimating the numbers of synonymous and nonsynonymous nucleotide substitutions. *Mol. Biol. Evolut.* **1986**, *3*, 418–426.

35. Andrews, R.M.; Kubacka, I.; Chinnery, P.F.; Lightowlers, R.N.; Turnbull, D.M.; Howell, N. Reanalysis and revision of the Cambridge reference sequence for human mitochondrial DNA. *Nat. Genet.* **1999**, *23*, 147. [CrossRef] [PubMed]

36. Krause, J.; Fu, Q.; Good, J.M.; Viola, B.; Shunkov, M.V.; Derevianko, A.P.; Pääbo, S. The complete mitochondrial DNA genome of an unknown hominin from southern Siberia. *Nature* **2010**, *464*, 894–897. [CrossRef] [PubMed]

37. Meyer, M.; Fu, Q.; Aximu-Petri, A.; Glocke, I.; Nickel, B.; Arsuaga, J.L.; Pääbo, S. A mitochondrial genome sequence of a hominin from Sima de los Huesos. *Nature* **2014**, *505*, 403–419. [CrossRef] [PubMed]

38. Green, R.E.; Malaspinas, A.S.; Krause, J.; Briggs, A.W.; Johnson, P.L.; Uhler, C.; Prüfer, K. A complete Neandertal mitochondrial genome sequence determined by high-throughput sequencing. *Cell* **2008**, *134*, 416–426. [CrossRef] [PubMed]

39. Sazonova, M.A.; Zhelankin, A.V.; Barinova, V.A.; Sinyov, V.V.; Khasanova, Z.B.; Postnov, A.Y.; Orekhov, A.N. Dataset of mitochondrial genome variants associated with asymptomatic atherosclerosis. *Data Brief.* **2016**, *7*, 1570–1575. [CrossRef] [PubMed]

40. Schultz, B.; Chan, S. Structures and proton-pumping strategies of mitochondrial respiratory enzymes. *Ann. Rev. Biophys. Biomol. Struct.* **2001**, *30*, 23–65. [CrossRef]

41. Hunte, C.; Koepke, J.; Lange, C.; Roßmanith, T.; Michel, H. Structure at 2.3 A resolution of the cytochrome bc (1) complex from the yeast *Saccharomyces cerevisiae* co-crystallized with an antibody Fv fragment. *Structure* **2000**, *8*, 669–684. [CrossRef]

42. Dasgupta, S.; Hoque, M.O.; Upadhyay, S.; Sidransky, D. Forced Cytochrome B gene mutation expression induces mitochondrial proliferation and prevents apoptosis in human uroepithelial SV-HUC-1 cells. *Int. J. Cancer* **2009**, *15*, 2829–2835. [CrossRef]

43. Mirabel, M.; Ferreira, B.; Sidi, D.; Lachaud, M.; Jouven, X.; Marijon, E. Rhumatisme articulaire aigu-Perspectives. *Med. Sci.* **2012**, *28*, 633–638.

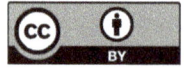

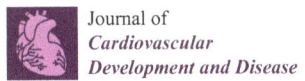

Journal of
Cardiovascular
Development and Disease

Article

Arterial Structural and Functional Characteristics at End of Early Childhood and Beginning of Adulthood: Impact of Body Size Gain during Early, Intermediate, Late and Global Growth

Juan M. Castro [1,†], Victoria García-Espinosa [1], Agustina Zinoveev [1], Mariana Marin [1], Cecilia Severi [2], Pedro Chiesa [3], Daniel Bia [1,†] and Yanina Zócalo [1,*,†]

1   Departamento de Fisiología, Facultad de Medicina, Centro Universitario de Investigación, Innovación y Diagnóstico Arterial, Universidad de la República, General Flores 2125, 11800 Montevideo, Uruguay
2   Departamento de Medicina Preventiva y Social, Instituto de Higiene, Facultad de Medicina, Universidad de la República, Alfredo Navarro 3051, 11600 Montevideo, Uruguay
3   Servicio de Cardiología Pediátrica, Centro Hospitalario Pereira-Rossell, ASSE-Facultad de Medicina, Universidad de la República, Bulevar Artigas 1550, 11600 Montevideo, Uruguay
*   Correspondence: yana@fmed.edu.uy; Tel.: +598-29243414-3313
†   These authors contributed equally to this work.

Received: 22 July 2019; Accepted: 21 August 2019; Published: 6 September 2019

Abstract: An association between nutritional characteristics in theearlylife stages and the state of the cardiovascular (CV) system in early childhood itself and/or at the beginning of adulthood has been postulated. It is still controversial whether changes in weight, height and/or body mass index (BMI) during childhood or adolescence are independently associated with hemodynamics and/or arterial properties in early childhood and adulthood. Aims: First, to evaluate and compare the strength of association between CVproperties (at 6 and 18 years (y)) and (a) anthropometric data at specific growth stages (e.g., birth, 6 y, 18 y) and (b) anthropometric changes during early (0–2 y), intermediate (0–6 y), late (6–18 y) and global (0–18 y) growth. Second, to determine whether the associations between CVproperties and growth related body changes depend on size at birth and/or at the time of CVstudy. Third, to analyze the capacity of growth-related body size changes to explain hemodynamic and arterial properties in early childhood and adulthood before and after adjusting for exposure to CV risk factors. Anthropometric, hemodynamic (central, peripheral) and arterial parameters (structural, functional; elastic, transitional and muscular arteries) were assessed in two cohorts (children, $n = 682$; adolescents, $n = 340$). Data wereobtained and analyzed following identical protocols. Results: Body-size changes in infancy (0–2 y) and childhood (0–6 y) showed similar strength of association with CV properties at 6 y. Conversely, 0–6, 6-18 or 0–18 ychanges were not associated with CV parameters at 18 y. The association between CV properties at 6 yand body-size changes during growth showed: equal or greater strength than the observed for body-size at birth, and lower strength compared to that obtained for current z-BMI. Conversely, only z-BMI at 18 y showed associations with CV z-scores at 18 y. Body size at birth showed almost no association with CVproperties at 6 or 18 y. Conclusion: current z-BMI showed the greatest capacity to explain variations in CV properties at 6 and 18 y. Variations in some CV parameters were mainly explained by growth-related anthropometric changes and/or by their interaction with current z-BMI. Body size at birth showed almost no association with arterial properties at 6 or 18 y.

Keywords: adolescents; arterial stiffness; birth weight; body-size trajectories; cardio-metabolic health; children; growth; intima-media thickness; blood pressure

---

1. Introduction

Childhood overweight or obesity have beenshown to be associated with an increase in the prevalence of cardiovascular risk factors (CRFs), cardiovascular (CV) risk and development of CV and metabolic diseases later in life [1–3]. This, together with the observed increase in the prevalence of obesity during childhood has led to an increased interest in knowing the factors associated with increased adiposity gain and the link between adiposity gain in early life-stages and future CV alterations; fundamental steps to enable the development of adequate prevention, control and/or treatment strategies. Several studies have been carried out in children and adolescents mainly with the aim of analyzing the association between hemodynamic or arterial characteristics in childhood or adolescence and: (1) body size at birth, (2) growth-related increases in body weight (BW), height (BH), BW-for-BH (BWH), and/or body mass index (BMI), and/or (3) body size at the time of CV evaluation. Results have been heterogeneous. Up to now the factors associated with body size gain as well as the mechanisms underlying the association (impact) of body characteristics and their growth-related changes with CV parameters are not fully known. The controversial findings and lack of a clear understanding of the problem could be attributed to its inherent complexity (e.g., age-related differential impact of body size gain, interaction among co-factors, dependence on prior anthropometric conditions), as well as to characteristics and differences between studies designed to address it (e.g., methodological approaches, publication bias, statistical analyses) [4–6].

Early accelerated BW gain (e.g., defined as an increase in BW-for-age z-score of at least 0.67 units between 0 and 2 years old (y)) would be associated with detrimental CV changes in children and adolescents [7,8]. In this regard, at least five interrelated issues should be clarified. First, the strength of the association between CV characteristics (i.e., hemodynamic and arterial) and anthropometric changes (e.g., early BW gain), along with their independence from birth weight and current body conditions.An association between low birth weight (LBW) and CV alterationshas been described, which would be reinforced by (or could even depend on) an accelerated BW gain in the postnatal period and/or by associated excessive subsequent adipose gain expressed by an elevated BMI at the time of CV evaluation [9]. Second, the magnitude of the interactions of anthropometric and CV parameters respect to body size at birth and current BMI should be addressed [10]. Third, the association between BW gain and CV parameters should be analyzed considering that it may depend on the timing of growth-related body changes (e.g., acceleration) [7,8] and/or on thesubject'sage (i.e., at the time of CVassessment) [6,11]. Fourth, as previous works reported that early growthpatterns could be associated with the development or exposure to factors associated with increased CV risk (CRFs' clustering) [12], the real (independent) clinical meaning or CV impact of BW gain should be determined, taking into account the exposure to CRFs. Fifth, the association between body size gain, birth-size and/or current anthropometric conditions with hemodynamic or arterial parameters could vary, depending on the: (a) arterial type (e.g., muscular vs. elastic); (b) site of evaluation and hemodynamic parameters considered (e.g., peripheral vs. central); and (c) arterial pathway considered (e.g., conductance vs. resistance) [13,14]. Recently, our group demonstrated that z-BMI variations in children and adolescents are positively associated with peripheral (brachial) and central (aortic) blood pressure levels (pBP and cBP, respectively); carotid, femoral and brachial artery diameters; carotid (but not femoral or brachial) intima-media thickness (IMT); arterial stiffness and stiffness gradient. Moreover, we found a "hierarchical order" among hemodynamic and arterial variations associated with z-BMI. pBP was the variable with the greatest variations associated with z-BMI (particularly pBP rather than cBP was associated with z-BMI). The stiffness of central (but not peripheral) arteries was associated with z-BMI (a pBP-dependent association). In turn, variations in arterial diameters were associated with z-BMI, without differences between the elastic and muscular arteries [13]. The above highlights the importance of a comprehensive, multiparametric approach when evaluating the CV system. If results obtained in an arterial segment and/or for a given parameter were generalized, significant errors (biases) could be made.

This work's aims were: (1) to evaluate and compare the strength of association between hemodynamic and arterial characteristics and (a) anthropometric data at specific growth stages (e.g., birth, 6 y, 18 y) and (b) body size changes during early (e.g., 0–2 y), intermediate (0–6 y), late (6–18 y) and global (0–18 y) growth; (2) to determine whether the association between CV characteristics and growth-related body size changes depends on size at birth and/or at the time of CV evaluation; and (3) to analyze the explanatory capacity of growth-related body size changes for hemodynamic and arterial characteristics in early childhood (6 y) and at the beginning of adulthood (18 y), before and after adjusting for body-size at birth, current BMI and/or exposure to CRFs.

2. Materials and Methods

2.1. Study Population

The study was carried out in the context of the Centro Universitario de Investigación, Innovación y Diagnóstico Arterial (CUiiDARTE) Project [13–16]. The protocol was approved by the Institutional Ethics Committee. Both parents' consent and child's assent were received before data collection. Participants (or their guardians) signed a written consent prior to the evaluation. Subjects from two cohorts, one of children (*n* = 682) and the other of adolescents (*n* = 340) were included (Table 1). The children cohort, defined based on probabilistic, bi-stage and stratified sampling of subjects attending public kindergartens in Montevideo, is part (subsample) of the longitudinal study "Patrón de crecimiento, estadonutricional y calidad de la alimentaciónen la primerainfancia: análisis de suimpactosobre la estructura y función vascular y el riesgo cardiovascular relativoenniñosuruguayos (CUiiDARTE-Agencia Nacional de Investigación e Innovación(ANII), Ministerio de Desarrollo Social (MIDES), United Nations Children's Fund(UNICEF) that started in 2010 (first phase) and had in 2016 a second phase [15,16]. In turn, the adolescent cohort (subsample from Montevideo) belongs to a longitudinal (four stages) study called "Estudio Longitudinal del Bienestaren Uruguay" (ELBU) aimed at investigating multidimensional well-being [17] working with a national representative sample of children (and their families) attending in 2004 the first grade of primary public schools in urban areas, which account for 87% of the Uruguayan population.

Similar approaches were carried out on children and adolescents: clinical and anthropometric evaluation, compilation (questionnaires) of data about lifestyle and family history (e.g., educational level, socioeconomic conditions, nutritional factors) and non-invasive CV evaluation.

2.2. Anthropometric Evaluation

Anthropometric data (BW and BH) corresponding to ages ≤36 months (mos.) were obtained from registers of the obligatory health-controlsfor children within those ages, established by the Ministry of Health (Children cohort). BW and length at birth in the adolescent cohort were obtained by documented self-report, during parents' interviews. In turn, following standard procedures, trained technicians obtained anthropometric data from children and adolescents (at participants' home, school and/or during the CV evaluation). BW and BH were measured with lightweight clothing and without shoes. Standing BH was measured (subject's head in the Frankfurt Plane position) using a portable stadiometer and recorded to the nearest 0.1 cm. BW was measured with an electronic scale (model 841/843, Seca Inc., Hamburg, Germany; model HBF-514C, Omron Inc., Chicago, Illinois, USA) and recorded to the nearest 0.1 kg. Two measurements were made and a third measurement was obtained in case the first two readings differed by more than 0.5 cm or 0.5 kg. After aggregating records from our technicians and those from health-controls, we obtained BW and BH data corresponding to: (1) birth, 6, 12, 18, 24, 36 and ~72 mos (~6 y) in the children cohort, and (2) birth, ~6 y, ~8 y, ~12 y and ~18 y in the adolescents' cohort. BMI was calculated as BW-to-squared BH ratio and converted into z-scores (z-BMI). Standardized z-scores for BMI and BWH (up to 2 y), BW-for-age, BH-for-age and BMI-for-age were obtained using World Health Organization software (Anthro-v.3.2.2; Anthro-Plus-v.1.0.4). The changes or differences (Δ) in BWH z-score (ΔBWH z-score) between birth (0 y) and 24 mos. (0–2y, children cohort) were determined. In turn, the changes in z-BMI (ΔBMI z-score) between 0 and 6 y (0–6y, both cohorts), 0 and 18 y (0–18y, adolescents cohort) and 6 and 18 y (6–18y, adolescents cohort) were calculated. Changes were always determined as the difference between the latest (e.g., 18 y) and the earliest (e.g., 0 y) z-score.

Table 1. Clinical, anthropometric and arterial parameters, of children and adolescent cohorts.

	Children Cohort (*n* = 632)						Adolescent Cohort (*n* = 340)					
	MV	STD	Min.	p25th	p75th	Max.	MV	STD	Min.	p25th	p75th	Max.
Demographic, anthropometric and cardiovascular risk factors												
Age (years)	6.02	0.3	5.07	5.80	6.26	6.66	18.2	0.50	17.0	17.8	18.5	20.7
Subjects (n, %female)	632 (49.5)						340 (53.2)					
Body weight (kg)	22.31	4.67	14.00	19.20	24.35	46.50	64.4	14.2	40.2	55.0	70.0	120.0
Body height (m)	1.14	0.05	0.99	1.10	1.17	1.33	1.66	0.09	1.32	1.60	1.73	1.94
BMI (Kg/m^2)	17.03	2.48	12.10	15.37	18.06	27.15	23.17	4.47	15.1	20.2	24.7	48.2
z-BMI (STD)	0.96	1.47	−2.60	0.06	1.62	7.37	0.36	1.16	-3.4	−0.4	1.0	4.8
z-BW for age (STD)	0.45	1.30	−2.39	−0.45	1.18	6.15	-	-	-	-	-	-
z-BH for age (STD)	−0.33	1.04	−3.43	−1.05	0.29	3.55	−0.41	0.88	−4.73	-0.90	0.13	2.39
Obesity (n, %)	108 (17.1)						26 (7.4)					
Dyslipidemia (n, %)	1 (0.2)						18 (5.3)					
Diabetes (n, %)	1 (0.2)						0 (0.0)					
Hypertension (n, %)	27 (4.3)						18 (5.3)					
CV Family background (n, %)	0 (0.0)						13 (3.9)					
Current Smoke (n, %)	0 (0.0)						35 (10.4)					
Anthropometric z-scores												
z-BW for age at birth (STD)	0.02	0.95	−5.24	−0.56	0.68	2.95	−0.18	1.24	−5.19	−0.89	0.57	2.87
z-BH for age at birth (STD)	−0.27	1.13	−4.91	−1.00	0.46	4.75	−0.35	1.52	−5.75	−1.15	0.46	4.82
z-BMI for age at birth (STD)	0.27	1.06	−3.59	−0.38	0.93	3.65	−0.01	1.72	−6.31	−1.00	0.96	5.56
z-BW for height 24 m. (STD)	0.59	1.26	−3.86	−0.20	1.29	4.76	-	-	-	-	-	-
z-BW for age 24 m. (STD)	0.38	1.14	−2.83	−0.44	1.08	4.54	-	-	-	-	-	-
z-BH for age 24 m. (STD)	−0.15	1.11	−4.12	−0.92	0.60	3.30	-	-	-	-	-	-
z-BMI for age 24 m. (STD)	0.66	1.29	−4.07	−0.15	1.40	5.42	-	-	-	-	-	-
1st Wave: anthropometry												
Age (years)	-	-	-	-	-	-	6.7	0.5	5.42	6.32	6.92	8.98
z-BW for age (STD)	-	-	-	-	-	-	0.39	1.01	−1.93	−0.27	1.06	3.56
z-BH for age (STD)	-	-	-	-	-	-	−0.13	0.93	−3.19	−0.72	0.53	2.10
z-BMI for age (STD)	-	-	-	-	-	-	0.65	0.99	−1.81	−0.08	1.27	4.63
2nd Wave: anthropometry												
Age (years)	-	-	-	-	-	-	8.1	0.4	6.82	7.77	8.38	10.27
z-BW for age (STD)	-	-	-	-	-	-	0.44	1.14	−2.40	−0.36	1.24	4.05
z-BH for age (STD)	-	-	-	-	-	-	−0.10	0.98	−4.53	−0.69	0.51	2.07
z-BMI for age (STD)	-	-	-	-	-	-	0.66	1.16	−3.12	−0.17	1.36	4.99
3rd Wave: anthropometry												
Age (years)	-	-	-	-	-	-	12.2	0.5	10.74	11.83	12.46	14.80
z-BW for age (STD)	-	-	-	-	-	-	-	-	-	-	-	-
z-BH for age (STD)	-	-	-	-	-	-	−0.03	1.12	−3.46	−0.87	0.71	2.98
z-BMI for age (STD)	-	-	-	-	-	-	0.47	1.14	−3.17	−0.37	1.23	3.12
Aortic and peripheral blood pressure, hemodynamic and wave reflection parameters												
Heart rate (beats/min)	91	11	66	84	99	134	69	12	43	61	76	132
pSBP (mmHg)	100	8	80	94	105	126	120	11	90	113	127	156
pDBP (mmHg)	59	7	50	54	62	86	64	7	48	60	68	100
pPP (mmHg)	41	7	24	36	46	77	56	11	21	48	63	90
pMBP (mmHg)	72	7	31	68	77	96	83	7	65	78	87	118
cSBP (mmHg)	83	6	64	78	87	100	102	9	83	96	107	135
cPP (mmHg)	22	4	7	19	25	43	37	8	18	31	43	61
CO (liter/min)	4.4	0.3	3.2	4.1	4.8	5.7	5.4	0.7	3.9	4.9	5.9	7.1
C.I. (liter/min/m^2)	4.9	0.6	3.5	4.4	5.4	5.9	3.2	0.8	1.8	2.9	3.5	16.0
SVR (s.mmHg/mL)	1.10	0.10	0.86	1.04	1.19	1.41	1.05	0.15	0.78	0.93	1.16	1.47
AIx (%)	9.7	9.7	−16	3	17	37	−0.7	9.1	−28.0	−6	5	25
AIx@75 (%)	17.0	9.3	−10	11	23	43	−3.3	10.0	−34.0	−10	2	27
AP (mmHg)	2	2	−5	1	4	9	−1	4	−15	−2	2	8
PF (mmHg)	20	5	7	17	23	43	36	10	9	29	42	82
PB (mmHg)	10	4	3	9	11	78	14	3	4	12	16	26

Table 1. *Cont.*

	Children Cohort (*n* = 632)						Adolescent Cohort (*n* = 340)					
	MV	STD	Min.	p25th	p75th	Max.	MV	STD	Min.	p25th	p75th	Max.
Structural arterial parameters, local and regional arterial stiffness												
R-CCA SD (mm)	6.04	0.50	4.83	5.70	6.39	7.41	6.82	0.51	5.20	6.48	7.11	8.82
R-CCA DD (mm)	5.38	0.47	4.21	5.03	5.71	6.91	6.16	0.47	4.53	5.88	6.46	7.90
R-CCA IMT (mm)	0.421	0.028	0.370	0.405	0.431	0.537	0.494	0.039	0.380	0.473	0.512	0.631
L-CCA SD (mm)	5.92	0.46	4.84	5.59	6.22	7.48	6.75	0.46	5.46	6.41	7.07	8.18
L-CCA DD (mm)	5.25	0.43	4.25	4.96	5.53	6.99	6.11	0.44	4.90	5.76	6.40	7.56
L-CCA IMT (mm)	0.420	0.027	0.316	0.405	0.431	0.567	0.492	0.042	0.343	0.472	0.508	0.722
R-CFA SD (mm)	4.74	0.53	3.44	4.42	5.05	6.50	7.20	0.99	5.42	6.44	7.94	9.76
R-CFA DD (mm)	4.42	0.51	3.13	4.11	4.72	6.11	6.87	0.93	5.22	6.13	7.52	9.44
R-CFA IMT (mm)	0.331	0.032	0.282	0.313	0.346	0.411	0.409	0.063	0.320	0.373	0.448	0.645
L-CFA SD (mm)	4.72	0.50	3.51	4.36	5.01	6.37	7.30	1.02	4.69	6.48	8.08	10.26
L-CFA DD (mm)	4.40	0.50	3.29	4.06	4.71	5.98	6.97	0.98	4.48	6.18	7.68	9.75
L-CFA IMT (mm)	0.335	0.026	0.271	0.319	0.355	0.398	0.393	0.060	0.313	0.355	0.417	0.585
R-CCA EM (mmHg)	187	45	71	156	216	304	360	89	181	292	416	643
L-CCA EM (mmHg)	179	46	54	146	205	314	358	88	186	300	397	670
R-CFA EM (mmHg)	618	267	237	417	724	1555	1317	530	533	944	1565	3411
L-CFA EM (mmHg)	592	219	219	427	711	1561	1349	535	529	962	1639	3497
cfPWV (m/s)	4.81	0.76	2.88	4.28	5.25	7.72	6.10	0.75	4.02	5.61	6.57	8.20

MV: mean value. STD: standard deviation. Min., Max.: minimum and maximum values. z: z-score. p25th, p75th: percentile 25 and 75. BW, BH: body weight and height. BMI: body mass index. CV: cardiovascular. pSBP, pDBP, pPP, pMBP: peripheral systolic, diastolic, pulse and mean pressure. CO, C.I.: cardiac output and index. cSBP, cPP: central systolic and pulse pressure. SVR: systemic vascular resistances. AIx, AIx@75: aortic augmentation index without and with heart rate adjustment. AP: augmented pressure. PF and PB: forward and backward aortic pressure component. R: Right. L: Left. CCA, CFA: common carotid and femoral artery. DD, SD: diastolic and systolic diameter. EM: elastic modulus. IMT: intima-media thickness. cfPWV: carotid-femoral pulse wave velocity.

2.3. Clinical Evaluation

None of the included subjects were taking medications, had congenital, chronic or infectious diseases at the moment of the CV study A brief clinical interview, together with the anthropometric evaluation enabled to assess CRFs exposure. Hypertension, dyslipidemia and diabetes were considered present if they had been previously diagnosed, in agreement with reference guidelines [18]. Subjects <16 y who had brachial systolic and/or diastolic pBP (pSBP and pDBP) >95th percentile for sex, age and BH during the study were considered with high BP levels (HBP); regardless previous diagnosis of hypertension. For subjects aged ≥16 y, HBP levels were defined using cutoff values similar to those for adults (pSBP ≥ 140 mmHg, pDBP ≥ 90 mmHg) [18]. Smokingwas defined as at least one cigarette/week for as long as a month. A family history of CV disease (CVD) was defined by presence of first-degree relatives with premature (<55 y in males; <65 y in females) CVD.

2.4. Cardiovascular Evaluation

CV studies were performed in children and adolescents (6 and 18 y, respectively) at the educational centers and/or in CUiiDARTE non-invasive vascular laboratories. The same protocol was applied in both cohorts (Figure 1) and was performed by experienced technicians using the same equipment. In order to reach steady hemodynamic conditions, before starting CV evaluation the subjects hada 10 min rest in a supine position in a quiet, temperature-controlled room.

2.5. Peripheral and Central Pressure and Aortic Wave-Derived Parameters

Heart rate (HR), pSBP and pDBP were obtained at 5 min intervals (Hem-4030, OmronInc., Illinois, USA). Peripheral pulse pressure (pPP = pSBP − pDBP) and mean BP (MBP = pDBP + pPP/3) were calculated. To assess cBP and aortic wave-derived parameters, radial artery BP waveforms were recorded using applanation tonometry (SphygmoCor-CvMS, AtCor-Medical, Sidney Australia) (Figure 1). Pressure signals were calibrated topDBP and MBP. A generalized transfer-function (GTF) enabled us to obtain the correspondingcBP waves and central systolic, diastolic and pulse pressure levels (cSBP, cDBP, cPP) [15,19] (Figure 1). Only adequate waveforms (visual inspection) and high-quality recordings (operator index ≥85) were considered. By means of pulse wave analysis (PWA) the first (P1) and second (P2) peaks in cBP wave were identified and their height (amplitude) and time were determined. Then, the difference between P2 and P1 was computed as central augmented pressure (AP) and used to quantify central aortic augmentation index (Aix = AP/cPP). Since AIx depends on HR, AIx adjusted to a 75 beats/minHR (AIx@75) was calculated. Forward and backward (Pf and Pb) components of the aortic pulse wave were also quantified (Figure 1). AIx is a measure of the contribution of reflections to cBP wave amplitude. It depends on the timing and magnitude of the reflected (backward) wave and is influenced by the compliance and structure of vessels distal to the site of measurement, as well as by the distance to the reflection sites. Greater Pb and/or AIx values indicate increased reflections and/or earlier return of reflected waves due to increased arterial stiffness and/or closer reflection sites. Systemic vascular resistance, cardiac output and index were quantified from brachial pulse contour analysis (Mobil-O-Graph, I.E.M.-GmbH, Stolberg, Germany) [15,19]. Only high quality records (index ≤2) and satisfactory waves (visual inspection) were considered. Subjects' values are the average of at least six consecutive records obtained in a single visit.

2.6. Arterial Beat-to-Beat Diameter and Intima-Media Thickness (IMT)

Left and right common carotid and femoral arteries (CCA, CFA) were analyzed using ultrasound (6–13 MHz, M-Turbo, SonoSite Inc., Bothell, WA, USA) and image sequences (30 s, B-Mode, longitudinal views) were stored for off-line analysis. Beat-to-beat diameter waves were obtained using border detection software. Systolic (SD) and end-diastolic (DD) diameters and IMT (far wall, end-diastolic) values were obtained averaging at least 20 beats (Figure 1). CCA diameter and IMT were measured one centimeter proximal to the bulb; CFA diameter and IMT were measured in the straight segment of the penultimate centimeter proximal to the arterial bifurcation (Figure 1) [13].

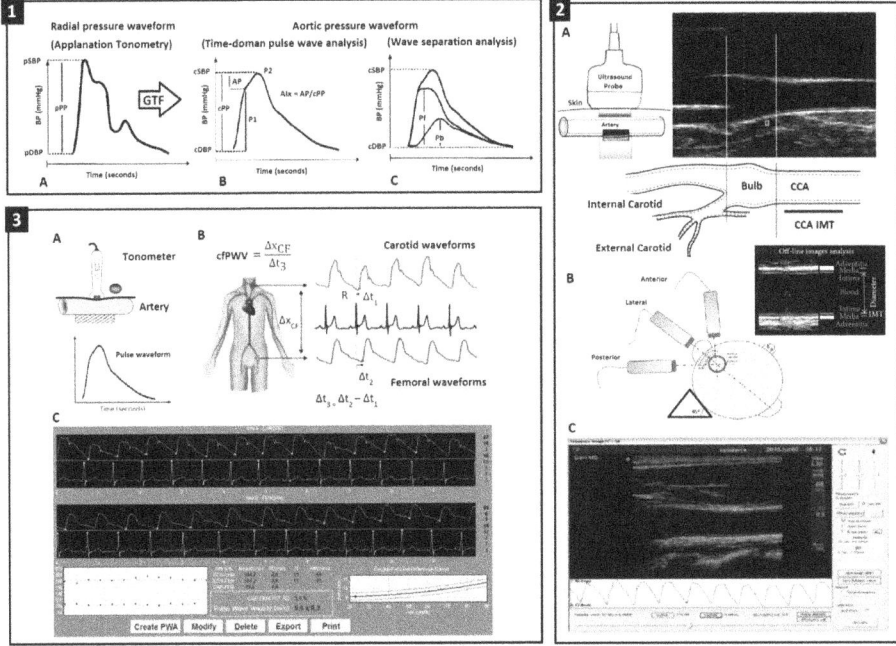

Figure 1. 1-A: Radial pulse wave obtained by applanation tonometry (SphygmoCor device); pSBP, pDBP, pPP: peripheral systolic, diastolic and pulse pressure. GTF: general transfer function. 1-B: Aortic wave derived using a GTF; augmented pressure (AP) and augmentation index (AIx) quantified from time-domain pulse wave analysis (PWA). cSBP, cDBP, cPP: central systolic, diastolic and pulsepressure. P1, P2: first and second pressure wave peaks. 1-C: Forward (Pf) and backward (Pb) components' amplitude obtained from wave separation analysis (WSA). 2-A, 2-B: Methodological approach used to assess common carotid (CCA) and femoral (CFA) artery diameter and intima-media thickness (IMT). Z: acoustic impedance. 2-C: Software for IMT and diameter measurement (Hemodyn-4M). 3-A, 3-B: Methodological approach used to assess carotid-femoral pulse wave velocity (cfPWV). Δx: CCA-to-CFA distance. Δt1, Δt2: time delay between R (ECG) and CCA and CFA foot wave. Δt3: time delay between arterial waves. 3-C: Software for cfPWV measurement (SphygmoCor device).

2.7. Local and Regional Arterial Stiffness

CCA and CFA pressure-strain elastic modulus (EM; local stiffness) were calculated as EM = PP/(SD − DD)/DD; cPP and pPP were considered to quantify CCA EM and CFA EM, respectively. Aortic regional stiffness was assessed by means of carotid-femoral pulse wave velocity (cfPWV) (SphygmoCor-CvMS) (Figure 1). The SphygmoCor allowed us to obtain cfPWV from sequential CCA and CFA wave recordings. cfPWV was calculated as the quotient between pulse wave travel distanceand pulse transit time. Real cfPWV was obtained multiplying measured cfPWV by 0.8. cfPWV values were obtained as the mean of three measurements.

2.8. Data Analysis and Statistics

A step-wise analysis was performed. First, CV variables were standardized and expressed as z-scores. To this end, subjects not exposed to CRFs (i.e., hypertension, HBP, dyslipidemia, smoking, diabetes, obesity or family history of CVD) were selected from each cohort (reference subgroups: 400 children, 153 adolescents) (Supplementary (S) Table S1). Working with the reference subgroups, mean value (MV) and standard deviation (STD) were determined for each variable (considering age and sex). Then, individual data were converted into z-scores (dimensionless numbers obtained by subtracting the reference MV from an observation, dividing the result by the reference STD) (Table S2) [13].

Second, Pearson product-moment correlations were obtained to quantify the strength of association between CVz-scores and anthropometric variables: (1) at birth: BWH z-score (both cohorts); (2) at the time of the CVstudy: current z-BMI (6 y for children, 18 y for adolescents); (3) growth-related changes: (a) early: ΔBWHz-score 0–2y, (b) intermediate: ΔBMI z-score 0–6y, (c) late: ΔBMI z-score 6–18y and (d) global: ΔBMI z-score 0–18y (Tables 2 and 3).

Third, statistical comparisons of the correlations' strengths were done using two-tailed William's test, making statistical corrections for dependent (same cohort) and overlapping (correlations have a variable in common) variables (e.g., when comparing the correlations "ΔBMI z-score 0–6y and z-pSBP" and "current z-BMI and z-pSBP" in the children cohort) [20] (Tables 2 and 3). Comparisons between cohorts were made considering William's test for non-overlapping (no variables in common) and independent (different cohort) variables (e.g., when comparing the R obtained for ΔBMI z-score 0–6y and z-pSBP in children and adolescents) (Table 4).

Fourth, the association between CV z-scores and anthropometric changes during growth was analyzed after statistical adjustment (partial correlations) for: (a) BWH z-score at birth; (b) BWH z-score at birth and current z-BMI and (c) BWH z-score at birth and ΔBMI z-score 6-18y (Tables 5–8). Multiple linear regression models (MLR; input: enter and forward), enabled to analyze the association between standardized CV data (dependent variables) and (1) single, specific anthropometric changes (ΔBWH z-score 0–2y, Δz-BMI 0–6y, Δz-BMI 0–18y and Δz-BMI 6–18y); (2) BWH z-score at birth; (3) current z-BMI, and (4) the interactions between growth-related changes and birth size or current z-BMI (e.g., (Δz-BMI 0–6y*BWH at birth) and (Δz-BMI 0–6y*current z-BMI)). In other words, since an association between postnatal growth and CV properties might be modified by birth or current body size, interaction between these conditions and growth-related body size changes on CV characteristics was tested adding two product terms (as continuous variables) to the model [21] (Tables S3–S12).

Fifth, using MLR models (input: enter and forward) we analyzed the association between standardized CV variables at 6 and 18 y and anthropometric variables and CRFs (independent variables) (Tables 8 and 9, Tables S13 and 14). A variance inflation factor (VIF) <5 was selected to evaluate (discard) significant collinearity.

Analyses were done using MedCalc Statistical Software (v.18.5. MedCalc Inc., Ostend, Belgium); Cocor Statistical Package (http://comparingcorrelations.org/) and IBM-SPSS Software (v.20, IBM-SPSS Inc., Chicago, IL, USA). A $p < 0.05$ was considered statistically significant.

3. Results

3.1. Arterial System at 6 and 18 y: Comparative Analysis of the Association between Birth or Current Body Size and Early, Intermediate, Late or Global Growth-Related Body Size Changes

The association between CV z-scores at 6 y and (a) body size at birth and 6 y or (b) body size changes during growing-up (0–2 or 0–6y) are shown in Table 2 (children cohort). Both, ΔBWH z-score 0–2y and Δz-BMI 0–6y, were associated with structural and hemodynamic parameters. Positive associations were found between z-pSBP, z-pMBP, z-cSBP, z-cDBP and the ΔBWH z-score 0–2y and Δ z-BMI 0-6y ($p < 0.05$). Negative associations were observed when z-AP, z-AIx and z-AIx@75 were considered. z-Pf was positively associated with Δz-BMI 0-6y (statistical threshold, $p = 0.053$), but the association with ΔBWH z-score 0–2 y did not reach significance ($p = 0.09$). The characteristics and statistical significance of the associations between anthropometric changes and structural properties varied, depending (among on other factors) on the structural parameter considered. No significant associations were found between stiffness z-scores and ΔBWH z-score 0-2 y and Δz-BMI 0–6 y (Table 2)

Table 2. Comparative analysis CV variables' association with anthropometric characteristics at birth, at 6 y and with anthropometric changes within that period (0–2 and 0–6 y) (children cohort, n = 632).

| | Zero-Order Correlations | | | | | | | | William Test (Comparison of Correlations) | | | | |
| | Δ z-BWH (0–2y) [1] | | Δ z-BMI (0–6y) [2] | | z-BWH (at Birth) [3] | | z-BMI (at 6 y) [4] | | 1–2 | 1–3 | 1–4 | 2–3 | 2–4 |
	R	p	R	p	R	p	R	p	p	p	p	p	p
Aortic and peripheral blood pressure, hemodynamic and wave reflection parameters													
z-pSBP	0.16	0.026	0.20	0.003	0.08	0.228	0.32	<0.001	0.408	0.469	0.019	0.245	0.009
z-pDBP	0.13	0.064	0.16	0.019	0.05	0.437	0.22	<0.001	0.538	0.476	0.182	0.299	0.174
z-pPP	0.05	0.474	0.06	0.389	0.03	0.613	0.13	0.034	0.839	0.883	0.236	0.805	0.110
z-pMBP	0.16	0.027	0.19	0.005	0.07	0.304	0.28	<0.001	0.514	0.425	0.062	0.243	0.038
z-cSBP	0.18	0.008	0.20	0.003	0.05	0.391	0.29	<0.001	0.663	0.253	0.079	0.138	0.042
z-cDBP	0.14	0.040	0.16	0.017	0.04	0.501	0.23	<0.001	0.665	0.355	0.150	0.237	0.091
z-cPP	0.06	0.396	0.07	0.312	0.04	0.579	0.10	0.106	0.831	0.831	0.549	0.726	0.534
z-AIx	-0.16	0.017	-0.17	0.009	0.11	0.078	-0.16	0.009	0.828	0.008	0.964	0.005	0.762
z-AIx@75	-0.16	0.020	-0.16	0.014	0.03	0.648	-0.23	<0.001	0.949	0.073	0.291	0.063	0.106
z-AP	-0.15	0.027	-0.14	0.030	0.12	0.054	-0.11	0.064	0.829	0.009	0.576	0.008	0.502
z-Pf	0.11	0.092	0.13	0.053	-0.02	0.791	0.17	0.006	0.667	0.208	0.427	0.143	0.395
z-Pb	0.01	0.938	0.00	0.949	0.04	0.494	0.03	0.609	0.850	0.709	0.701	0.634	0.427
Structural arterial parameters, local and regional arterial stiffness													
z-R-CCA SD	0.08	0.455	0.24	0.016	0.03	0.785	0.32	0.001	0.026	0.758	0.036	0.168	0.430
z-R-CCA DD	0.07	0.506	0.22	0.024	0.03	0.744	0.22	0.002	0.002	0.820	0.033	0.225	0.311
z-R-CCA IMT	-0.29	0.004	0.28	0.005	-0.05	0.631	0.13	<0.001	<0.001	0.018	<0.001	0.001	0.833
z-L-CCA SD	0.12	0.092	0.15	0.027	0.13	0.039	0.28	0.037	0.532	0.911	0.476	0.923	0.545
z-L-CCA DD	0.09	0.206	0.14	0.035	0.16	0.012	0.29	<0.001	0.298	0.469	0.003	0.812	<0.001
z-L-CCA IMT	0.11	0.115	0.14	0.043	0.07	0.178	0.29	0.004	0.695	0.735	0.312	0.513	0.390
z-R-CFA SD	0.32	0.003	0.36	<0.001	-0.16	0.118	0.18	<0.001	0.807	0.004	0.708	0.001	0.952
z-R-CFA DD	0.34	0.001	0.35	<0.001	-0.18	0.077	0.36	<0.001	0.827	0.002	0.890	0.001	0.765
z-R-CFA IMT	-0.23	0.338	-0.25	0.296	0.14	0.552	0.33	0.065	0.674	0.335	0.470	0.294	0.323
z-L-CFA SD	0.11	0.123	0.14	0.034	0.09	0.194	-0.40	<0.001	0.767	0.838	0.086	0.610	<0.001
z-L-CFA DD	0.09	0.198	0.12	0.071	0.08	0.208	0.29	<0.001	0.690	0.948	0.014	0.730	0.002
z-L-CFA IMT	0.08	0.617	0.17	0.250	-0.12	0.379	0.26	0.919	0.101	0.372	0.542	0.173	0.001
z-R-CCA EM	0.05	0.620	0.12	0.226	-0.02	0.822	-0.01	0.162	0.205	0.650	0.463	0.028	0.864
z-L-CCA EM	-0.03	0.746	0.06	0.405	0.11	0.161	0.13	0.080	0.242	0.280	0.057	0.697	0.213
z-R-CFA EM	0.15	0.179	0.07	0.493	-0.08	0.422	0.12	0.981	0.103	0.177	0.189	0.353	0.343
z-L-CFA EM	-0.04	0.596	-0.06	0.407	0.04	0.579	0.00	0.863	0.115	0.993	0.703	0.360	0.287
z-cfPWV	0.00	0.991	-0.03	0.775	-0.02	0.790	-0.01	1.00	0.649	0.876	0.989	0.959	0.610

z: z-score. BW, BH: body weight and height. Δ: change in the analyzed period. BMI: body mass index. SBP, DBP, PP, MBP: systolic, diastolic, pulse and mean pressure (p: peripheral, c: central). AIx, AIx@75: aortic augmentation index without and with heart rate adjustment. AP: augmented pressure. Pf, Pb: forward and backward pressure components. R: Right. L: Left. CCA, CFA: common carotid and femoral artery. EM: elastic modulus. IMT: intima-media thickness. DD, SD: diastolic and systolic diameter. cfPWV: carotid-femoral pulse wave velocity. R: Pearson coefficient. $p < 0.05$ (red text) was considered significant. In Zero-order correlations columns, the numbers in square brackets define de groups. Then in "William Test (Comparison of Correlations)" (also in columns in the same table), groups are compared in pairs cnsidering groups numbers. Identical comment for next Tables.

Unlike BWH at birth, current z-BMI (6y) was associated with hemodynamic and structural parameters. Furthermore, whereas BWH at birth did not show significant associations with hemodynamic variables, current z-BMI was associated ($p < 0.05$) with almost all of them (pBP, cBPandwave-derived parameters) (Table 2).

Compared to ΔBWH z-score 0–2y and Δz-BMI 0–6y, current z-BMI levels (at 6 y) were more strongly associated with CV z-scores. For example, R coefficients for the association between z-pSBP and ΔBWH z-score 0–2y, Δz-BMI 0–6y and current z-BMI (6 y) were 0.16, 0.20 and 0.32, respectively ($p < 0.05$). When compared, the association was stronger in case of z-BMI at 6 y ($p = 0.019$ and $p = 0.009$) (Table 2). The strength of association between arterial parameters at 6 y and ΔBWH z-score 0–2y and Δz-BMI 0–6y did not show statistical differences, with the only exception of z-Right CCA SD, DD and IMT that showed stronger association with 0–6y changes ($p = 0.026$, $p = 0.002$ and $p < 0.01$, respectively).

In adolescents, CVz-scores showed associations with current z-BMI, while almost no association was observed between arterial parameters at 18 y and prior body size characteristics (i.e., BWH at birth and Δz-BMI 0-6y) (Table 3). On the other hand, in case of variables associated with Δz-BMI 0–18y (z-pSBP, z-pPP, z-CCA SD and DD) or BWH z-score at birth (z-Right CCA EM and z-Left CCA EM), the comparative analysis (William's test) showed that the strongest associations were obtained when considering current z-BMI (18 y) (Table 3).

Jointly analyzing data from both cohorts it was observed that the strength of the associations between CV z-scores and current z-BMI (6 or 18 y), were always greater than those obtained for any change in body size between birth and the time of the study (0–2, 0–6 or 6–18 y) (Tables 2 and 3).

As mentioned, arterial properties at 6 y were associated with body size changes in that life period (i.e., 0–2 and 0–6 y) whereas the CV properties in subjects 18 y showed almost no association with prior (i.e., Δz-BMI 0–6, 6–18 and 0–18 y) anthropometric conditions (Table 4). When the cohorts were statistically compared, it was observed that for the same "body change" (Δz-BMI 0–6 y), associations were significant for almost all the studied variables when subjects were 6 y, but not when they were 18 y (Table 4).

Thus, as the subject's age increases, the association between CV z-scores and prior anthropometric changes (i.e., during childhood) decreases (Table 4).

3.2. Arterial Structure and Function at 6 y: Independent Association with ΔBWH z-Score 0–2 y

Associations between hemodynamic and structural parameters at 6 y and ΔBWH z-score 0–2 y kept significant after controlling for BWH z-score at birth (Table 5). After adjusting for BWH z-score at birth and current z-BMI only associations with z-cSBP (but not with z-pSBP, $p = 0.103$) remained significant ($R = 0.14$, $p = 0.041$) (Table 5). Thus, the association between ΔBWH z-score 0-2 y and cSBP, while weak, is independent of size at birth and at the time of CV study. AIx@75 ($p = 0.009$) and Pf ($p = 0.052$) showed significant associations after controlling for body size at birth (Table 5).

As mentioned, significant positive associations were found between ΔBWH z-score 0–2 y and structural parameters. Disregarding BWH z-scores at birth, ΔBWH z-score 0-2y values were positively associated with z-IMT (both CCA) and z-diameters (both CFA, left CCA). Then, the greater the body size change within the first 2 y, the higher the diameters and wall thickness (Table 5). The associations between ΔBWH z-score 0–2 y and z-IMT remained significant after adjusting for BWH at birth and current z-BMI (6 y). Then, regardless of nutritional status at birth and at the time of arterial evaluation, z-IMT levels at 6 y are influenced by ΔBWH z-score 0–2y (Table 5).

There were no significant associations between ΔBWH z-score 0–2 y and stiffness z-scores, before (zero-order correlations) and after (partial correlations) adjusting for BWH z-scores at birth and/or current z-BMI (Table 5).

Table 3. Comparative analysis CV variables' association with anthropometric characteristics at birth, at 18 y and with anthropometric changes within that period (0–6, 0–18, 6–18 y) [adolescent cohort, n = 340].

	Zero-Order correlations										William Test (Comparison of Correlations)								
	Δ z-BMI (0–6y) [1]		Δ z-BMI (0–18y) [2]		Δ z-BMI (6–18y) [3]		z-BWH (at Birth) [4]		z-BMI (18y) [5]		1-2	1-3	1-4	1-5	2-3	2-4	2-5	3-4	3-5
	R	p	R	p	R	p	R	p	R	p	p	p	p	p	p	p	p	p	p
Aortic and peripheral blood pressure, hemodynamic and reflection parameters																			
z-pSBP	0.08	0.234	0.14	0.021	0.09	0.172	0.01	0.931	0.25	<0.001	0.411	0.905	0.488	0.010	0.421	0.203	0.040	0.458	0.009
z-pDBP	-0.02	0.757	0.02	0.798	0.07	0.286	0.03	0.581	0.17	0.002	0.623	0.283	0.609	0.004	0.424	0.922	0.006	0.711	0.107
z-pPP	0.10	0.111	0.14	0.016	0.04	0.478	-0.02	0.715	0.15	0.007	0.541	0.473	0.002	0.460	0.108	0.118	0.854	0.579	0.077
z-pMBP	0.02	0.732	0.08	0.206	0.09	0.162	0.03	0.660	0.24	<0.001	0.438	0.403	0.954	0.001	0.873	0.283	0.003	0.577	0.014
z-cSBP	0.02	0.765	0.07	0.226	0.05	0.461	0.10	0.081	0.27	<0.001	0.464	0.721	0.421	<0.001	0.749	0.775	<0.001	0.641	0.000
z-cDBP	0.002	0.977	0.03	0.613	-0.01	0.818	0.09	0.135	0.14	0.011	0.692	0.886	0.396	0.038	0.523	0.568	0.050	0.353	0.016
z-cPP	0.02	0.773	0.05	0.394	0.06	0.301	0.04	0.504	0.18	0.001	0.663	0.634	0.844	0.017	0.873	0.924	0.020	0.853	0.053
z-AIx	0.02	0.744	0.02	0.682	0.03	0.602	-0.01	0.931	-0.02	0.774	0.944	0.906	0.495	0.008	0.874	0.772	0.471	0.714	0.428
z-AIx@75	-0.05	0.416	0.004	0.948	0.09	0.159	0.07	0.265	0.01	0.918	0.451	0.287	0.266	0.110	0.172	0.523	0.970	0.853	0.204
z-AP	0.02	0.735	0.02	0.741	0.02	0.744	0.001	0.996	-0.02	0.693	1.000	0.987	0.850	<0.001	0.992	0.849	0.470	0.398	0.526
z-PF	0.06	0.397	0.06	0.308	0.02	0.707	-0.02	0.755	0.11	0.047	0.967	0.643	0.459	0.432	0.535	0.449	0.376	0.719	0.161
z-PB	0.11	0.096	0.06	0.309	-0.08	0.211	0.05	0.402	0.06	0.289	0.519	0.028	0.578	0.484	0.030	0.925	0.990	0.243	0.030
Structural arterial parameters, local and regional arterial stiffness																			
z-R-CCA SD	0.09	0.146	0.15	0.015	0.10	0.123	-0.02	0.692	0.26	<0.001	0.437	0.905	0.273	0.012	0.423	0.098	0.041	0.269	0.009
z-R-CCA DD	0.08	0.208	0.14	0.021	0.09	0.129	-0.003	0.962	0.26	<0.001	0.413	0.905	0.291	0.006	0.424	0.164	0.026	0.392	0.006
z-R-CCA IMT	0.04	0.501	0.03	0.604	0.12	0.060	0.002	0.967	0.12	0.032	0.900	0.341	0.716	0.238	0.153	0.787	0.104	0.277	0.949
z-L-CCA SD	0.11	0.077	0.13	0.034	0.10	0.100	-0.01	0.883	0.25	<0.001	0.811	0.905	0.248	0.034	0.632	0.174	0.026	0.312	0.015
z-L-CCA DD	0.10	0.121	0.12	0.054	0.09	0.136	0.03	0.597	0.28	<0.001	0.822	0.905	0.513	0.007	0.632	0.382	0.003	0.581	0.002
z-L-CCA IMT	0.12	0.069	0.06	0.283	0.09	0.150	-0.01	0.868	0.13	0.020	0.440	0.721	0.212	0.860	0.634	0.772	0.205	0.359	0.524
z-R-CFA SD	0.12	0.233	0.08	0.418	0.18	0.057	0.02	0.840	0.34	<0.001	0.708	0.647	0.537	0.036	0.309	0.712	0.002	0.345	0.133
z-R-CFA DD	0.11	0.281	0.08	0.437	0.18	0.069	0.01	0.957	0.32	<0.001	0.755	0.593	0.522	0.046	0.309	0.667	0.004	0.316	0.140
z-R-CFA IMT	0.15	0.496	0.17	0.390	0.19	0.363	-0.16	0.423	0.27	0.149	0.936	0.886	0.380	0.607	0.924	0.343	0.582	0.339	0.697
z-L-CFA SD	0.11	0.292	0.11	0.244	0.11	0.273	-0.02	0.870	0.26	0.003	0.986	0.988	0.440	0.148	0.960	0.422	0.077	0.446	0.120
z-L-CFA DD	0.09	0.407	0.10	0.307	0.10	0.322	0.01	0.951	0.26	0.003	0.943	0.940	0.607	0.100	0.984	0.578	0.059	0.597	0.097
z-L-CFA IMT	0.01	0.967	-0.15	0.445	-0.26	0.190	0.27	0.162	0.33	0.068	0.160	0.328	0.437	0.151	0.589	0.215	0.005	0.136	0.002
z-R-CCA EM	-0.05	0.485	0.02	0.788	0.06	0.317	0.12	0.043	0.21	<0.001	0.360	0.196	0.102	<0.001	0.528	0.327	0.003	0.581	0.016
z-L-CCA EM	0.02	0.787	0.06	0.296	0.06	0.345	0.13	0.029	0.31	<0.001	0.551	0.639	0.288	<0.001	0.954	0.498	0.003	0.520	<0.001
z-R-CFA EM	-0.03	0.793	0.02	0.821	-0.10	0.308	-0.09	0.364	-0.07	0.443	0.648	0.601	0.725	0.721	0.230	0.503	0.306	0.953	0.764
z-L-CFA EM	-0.14	0.175	-0.05	0.630	-0.09	0.351	0.12	0.223	0.09	0.309	0.408	0.706	0.118	0.032	0.689	0.298	0.109	0.222	0.070
z-cfPWV	0.01	0.912	0.01	0.802	-0.03	0.621	0.03	0.632	0.03	0.599	0.944	0.633	0.862	0.770	0.523	0.845	0.716	0.579	0.337

z: z-score. BW, BH: body weight and height. Δ: change in the studied period. BMI: body mass index. SBP, DBP, PP, MBP: systolic, diastolic, pulse and mean pressure (p: peripheral, c: central). AIx, AIx@75: augmentation index without and with heart rate adjustment. AP: augmentation pressure. Pf, Pb: forward and backwardpressure components. R: Right. L: Left. CCA, CFA: common carotid and femoral artery. EM: elastic modulus. IMT: intima-media thickness. DD, SD: diastolic and systolic diameter. cfPWV: carotid-femoral pulse wave velocity. R: Pearson coefficient. $p < 0.05$ (red) was considered significant.

Table 4. Comparative analysis of the associations between CV and anthropometric parameters: children vs. adolescents.

| | Zero-Order Correlations | | | | | | | | | | Comparison of Correlations | | | | | |
| | Children Cohort (n = 632) | | | | Adolescent Cohort (n = 340) | | | | | | | | | | | |
	ΔBWH (0-2y) [1]		Δ z-BMI (0-6y) [2]		Δ z-BMI (0-6y) [3]		Δ z-BMI (0-18y) [4]		Δ z-BMI (6-18y) [5]		1-3	1-4	1-5	2-3	2-4	2-5
	R	p	R	p	R	p	R	p	R	p	p	p	p	p	p	p
Aortic and peripheral blood pressure, hemodynamic and wave reflection parameters																
z-pSBP	0.16	0.026	0.20	0.003	0.08	0.234	0.14	0.021	0.09	0.172	0.320	0.802	0.384	0.613	0.449	0.169
z-pDBP	0.13	0.064	0.16	0.019	−0.02	0.757	0.02	0.798	0.07	0.286	0.065	0.175	0.458	0.708	0.084	0.264
z-pPP	0.05	0.474	0.06	0.389	0.10	0.111	0.14	0.016	0.04	0.478	0.538	0.266	0.624	0.902	0.322	0.806
z-pMBP	0.16	0.027	0.19	0.005	0.02	0.732	0.08	0.206	0.09	0.162	0.083	0.320	0.383	0.705	0.170	0.211
z-cSBP	0.18	0.008	0.20	0.003	0.02	0.765	0.07	0.226	0.05	0.461	0.047	0.159	0.097	0.794	0.095	0.055
z-cDBP	0.14	0.040	0.16	0.017	0.002	0.977	0.03	0.613	−0.01	0.818	0.080	0.163	0.058	0.797	0.098	0.031
z-cPP	0.06	0.396	0.07	0.312	0.02	0.773	0.05	0.394	0.06	0.301	0.614	0.900	0.930	0.899	0.801	0.899
z-AIx	−0.16	0.017	−0.17	0.009	0.02	0.744	0.02	0.682	0.03	0.602	0.023	0.023	0.016	0.897	0.016	0.011
z-AIx@75	−0.16	0.020	−0.16	0.014	−0.05	0.416	0.004	0.948	0.09	0.159	0.169	0.041	0.002	0.962	0.041	0.002
z-AP	−0.15	0.027	−0.14	0.030	0.02	0.735	0.02	0.741	0.02	0.744	0.035	0.032	0.032	0.898	0.043	0.043
z-Pf	0.11	0.092	0.13	0.053	0.06	0.397	0.06	0.308	0.06	0.707	0.534	0.534	0.263	0.802	0.383	0.063
z-Pb	0.01	0.938	−0.004	0.949	0.11	0.096	0.06	0.309	−0.08	0.211	0.215	0.537	0.266	0.883	0.429	0.347
Structural arterial parameters, local and regional arterial stiffness																
z-R-CCA SD	0.08	0.455	0.24	0.016	0.09	0.146	0.15	0.015	0.10	0.123	0.924	0.503	0.248	0.121	0.377	0.173
z-R-CCA DD	0.07	0.506	0.22	0.024	0.08	0.208	0.14	0.021	0.09	0.129	0.924	0.404	0.849	0.148	0.435	0.208
z-R-CCA IMT	−0.29	0.004	0.28	0.005	0.04	0.501	0.03	0.604	0.12	0.060	0.001	0.002	<0.001	<0.001	0.015	0.115
z-L-CCA SD	0.12	0.092	0.15	0.027	0.11	0.077	0.13	0.034	0.10	0.100	0.900	0.900	0.803	0.706	0.801	0.530
z-L-CCA DD	0.09	0.206	0.14	0.035	0.10	0.121	0.12	0.054	0.09	0.136	0.901	0.708	0.940	0.531	0.802	0.531
z-L-CCA IMT	0.11	0.115	0.14	0.043	0.12	0.069	0.06	0.283	0.09	0.150	0.900	0.535	0.803	0.708	0.318	0.531
z-R-CFA SD	0.32	0.003	0.36	<0.001	0.12	0.233	0.08	0.418	0.18	0.057	0.100	0.050	0.244	0.725	0.021	0.129
z-R-CFA DD	0.34	0.001	0.35	0.001	0.11	0.281	0.08	0.437	0.18	0.069	0.058	0.033	0.180	0.930	0.026	0.153
z-R-CFA IMT	−0.23	0.338	−0.25	0.296	0.15	0.496	0.17	0.390	0.19	0.363	0.173	0.151	0.131	0.942	0.131	0.113
z-L-CFA SD	0.11	0.123	0.14	0.034	0.11	0.292	0.11	0.244	0.11	0.273	0.992	0.977	0.992	0.773	0.773	0.773
z-L-CFA DD	0.09	0.198	0.12	0.071	0.09	0.407	0.10	0.307	0.10	0.322	0.970	0.924	0.924	0.774	0.848	0.848
z-L-CFA IMT	0.08	0.617	0.17	0.250	0.01	0.967	−0.15	0.445	−0.26	0.190	0.751	0.296	0.118	0.679	0.145	0.048
z-R-CCA EM	0.05	0.620	0.12	0.226	−0.05	0.485	0.02	0.788	0.06	0.317	0.355	0.781	0.926	0.515	0.353	0.576
z-L-CCA EM	−0.03	0.746	0.06	0.405	0.02	0.787	0.06	0.296	0.06	0.345	0.570	0.306	0.306	0.306	0.991	0.955
z-R-CFA EM	0.15	0.179	0.07	0.493	−0.03	0.793	0.02	0.821	−0.10	0.308	0.160	0.309	0.051	0.530	0.698	0.186
z-L-CFA EM	−0.04	0.596	−0.06	0.407	−0.14	0.175	−0.05	0.630	−0.09	0.351	0.343	0.925	0.637	0.851	0.925	0.777
z-cfPWV	−0.001	0.991	−0.03	0.775	0.01	0.912	0.01	0.802	−0.03	0.621	0.908	0.9082	0.761	0.761	0.753	0.95

z: z-score. BW, BH: body weight and height. Δ: change in the analyzed period. BMI: body mass index. SBP, DBP, PP, MBP: systolic, diastolic, pulse and mean pressure (p: peripheral, c: central). AIx, AIx@75: aortic augmentation index without and with heart rate adjustment. AP: augmented pressure. Pf, Pb: forward and backward pressure components. R: Right. L: Left. CCA, CFA: common carotid and femoral artery. EM: elastic modulus. IMT: intima-media thickness. DD, SD: diastolic and systolic diameter. cfPWV: carotid-femoral pulse wave velocity. R: Pearson coefficient. $p < 0.05$ (red) was considered significant.

3.3. Arterial Structure and Function at 6 and 18 y: Independent Association with Δz-BMI(Body Mass Index) 0–6 y

Table 6 shows correlations between CV z-scores (at 6 and 18 y) and Δz-BMI 0-6y. In children, z-pSBP, z-pDBP, z-pMBP, z-cSBP, z-cDPB and z-cMBP correlated (positively) with Δz-BMI 0–6 y. Associations remained significant after controlling for BWH at birth, but showed dependence on current z-BMI. AIx and AIx@75 showed significant negative associations when controlling for BWH at birth but when controlling for z-BMI at 6 y, positive correlations were observed ($R=0.14$, $p = 0.034$; $R=0.19$, $p = 0.005$). Both z-CCA IMT were associated with Δz-BMI 0–6 y, with independence of BWH at birth and current z-BMI. Similar results were observed for right and left CFA IMT and DD.

CV parameters (z-scores) at 18 ywere not associated (zero-order correlation) with Δz-BMI 0–6 y. However, several correlations became significant after adjusting for BWH z-scores at birth. Then, body size changes within 0–6 y would contribute to explain CV characteristics at 18 y. Unlike the observed at 6 y, CVparameters at 18 ywere not associated with Δz-BMI 0–6 y (except z-Pb and z-left CCA IMT) after adjusting for body size at birth and current z-BMI (Table 6)

3.4. Arterial Structure and Function at 18 y: Independent Association with Δz-BMI 0–18 y and 6–18 y

Tables 7 and 8 show the association between CV z-scores and Δz-BMI 0–18 and 6–18 y. There were no independent associations between CV properties at 18 y and overall (0–18 y) or late (6–18 y) anthropometric (z-BMI) changes, being the only exceptions z-pPP (for Δz-BMI 0–18 y; $p = 0.017$) and z-Right CCA SD (for Δz-BMI 6–18 y; $p = 0.035$). Then, global changes in body size from birth (0–18 y) or childhood (6–18 y) until late in adolescence would not contribute to explain CV characteristics at the beginning of adulthood, with independence of birth size or current z-BMI.

3.5. Hemodynamic and Arterial Properties at 6 and 18 y: Hierarchical Impact of Anthropometric Variables

MLRmodels allowed analyzing whether growth-related body size changes contribute to explain CV properties, considering and comparing BWH z-score at birth, current z-BMI and the interaction of variables (Supplementary Tables S3–S12). In children, cBP and pBP variables (z-SBP, z-DBP, z-PP, z-MBP) were only explained by z-BMI, while wave-derived parameters were explained by z-BMI (z-AIx@75, z-Pf, z-Pb), ΔBWH z-score 0–2 y (z-AIx, z-AP), Δz-BMI 0–6 y (z-AIx) and by Δz-BMI 0–6 y and z-BMI interaction (z-AP). Structural variables were mainly explained by z-BMI; arterial stiffness showed no association with body size parameters (Supplementary Tables S3–S6).

In the adolescents: (1) Δz-BMI 0–6 y showed explanatory capacity when interacting with current z-BMI (both z-CFA IMT) (Supplementary Tables S7 and S8); (2) Δz-BMI 0–18 y showed explanatory capacity when interacting with current z-BMI (z-cDBP, z-Right CFA diameters) or BWH z-score at birth (z-cDBP, z-cPP) (Supplementary Tables S9 and S10) and (3) Δz-BMI 6–18 ydid not showsignificant explanatory capacity for the studied variables (Supplementary Tables S11 and S12). Current z-BMI was always the variable with the greatest explanatory power. The explanatory capacity of the interactions between z-BMI (or z-BWH at birth) and Δz-BMI 0-6, 0–18 or 6–18 y was limited. Compared to current z-BMI, intermediate (0–6 y), late (6–18 y) or global (0–18 y) body-size changes showed almost no explanatory capacityfor interindividual variations in CV properties at 18 y.

The joint analysis of both cohorts showed that CV variables were mainly associated with current (i.e., 6 or 18 y) z-BMI. Body-size changes showed little individual explanatory power and their contribution was mainly relatedto the interaction with z-BMI at the time of CVevaluation.

3.6. Arterial Function at 6 and 18 y: Impact of Body Size Changes vs. Anthropometric and Cardiovascular Risk Factors (CRFs)

Table 9 and Supplementary Table S13 show explanatory models for CV parameters in children. pBP parameters were explained by current z-BMI, while cBP parameters and wave-derivedindexes were mainly associated with z-pSBP. Then, early (0–2 y) or intermediate (0–6 y) body size changes contributed little to explain cBP or pBPvariations found at 6 y compared to the conditions associated with CV risk (i.e., BMI and pSBP) at the time of the CV study.

Table 5. Associations between CV z-scores and z-BWHvariations between 0–2y (childrencohort, $n = 632$).

			Δ z-BWH (0–2y)			
	Zero-Order		Partial [1]		Partial [2]	
	R	*p*	*R*	*p*	*R*	*p*
Aortic and peripheral blood pressure, hemodynamic and wave reflection parameters						
z-pSBP	0.16	0.026	0.26	<0.001	0.11	0.103
z-pDBP	0.13	0.064	0.21	0.003	0.10	0.136
z-pPP	0.05	0.474	0.09	0.197	0.02	0.756
z-pMBP	0.16	0.027	0.25	<0.001	0.12	0.082
z-cSBP	0.18	0.008	0.27	<0.001	0.14	0.041
z-cDBP	0.14	0.040	0.21	0.002	0.10	0.136
z-cPP	0.06	0.396	0.10	0.135	0.06	0.379
z-AIx	−0.16	0.017	−0.12	0.085	−0.02	0.797
z-AIx@75	−0.16	0.020	−0.18	0.009	−0.06	0.419
z-AP	−0.15	0.027	−0.09	0.167	−0.02	0.762
z-Pf	0.11	0.092	0.13	0.052	0.04	0.528
z-Pb	0.01	0.938	0.04	0.545	0.03	0.619
Structural arterial parameters, local and regional arterial stiffness						
z-R-CCA SD	0.08	0.455	0.12	0.250	−0.06	0.595
z-R- CCA DD	0.07	0.506	0.11	0.277	−0.06	0.569
z-R-CCA IMT	−0.29	0.004	0.34	0.001	0.27	0.008
z-L-CCA SD	0.12	0.092	0.26	<0.001	0.13	0.058
z-L-CCA DD	0.09	0.206	0.24	<0.001	0.12	0.088
z-L-CCA IMT	0.11	0.115	0.20	0.004	0.13	0.048
z-R-CFA SD	0.32	0.003	0.28	0.008	0.08	0.472
z-R-CFA DD	0.34	0.001	0.30	0.005	0.12	0.288
z-R-CFA IMT	−0.23	0.338	−0.19	0.451	0.07	0.777
z-L-CFA SD	0.11	0.123	0.21	0.003	0.07	0.353
z-L-CFA DD	0.09	0.198	0.18	0.009	0.05	0.453
z-L-CFA IMT	0.08	0.617	0.00	0.991	−0.01	0.956
z-R-CCA EM	0.05	0.620	0.05	0.644	−0.03	0.750
z-L-CCA EM	−0.03	0.746	0.05	0.528	−0.01	0.888
z-R-CFA EM	0.15	0.179	0.12	0.270	0.13	0.223
z-L-CFA EM	−0.04	0.596	−0.02	0.796	−0.01	0.888
z-cfPWV	0.00	0.991	−0.02	0.827	−0.03	0.766

z: z-score. BW, BH: body weight and height. BMI: body mass index. SBP, DBP, PP, MBP: systolic, diastolic, pulse and mean pressure (p: peripheral, c: central). AIx, AIx@75: aortic augmentation index without and with heart rate adjustment. AP: augmented pressure. Pf, Pb: forward and backward pressure components. CCA, CFA: common carotid and femoral artery. EM: elastic modulus. IMT: intima-media thickness. DD, SD: diastolic and systolic diameter. cfPWV: carotid-femoral pulse wave velocity. *R*: Pearson coefficient. $p < 0.05$ (red) was considered significant. Partial correlations controlling for: [1] BW-for-BH (length) z-score at birth; [2] BW-for-BH (length) z-score at birth and z-BMI at the time of measurement (6 y).

Table 6. Associations between CV z-scores and z-BMIvariations between 0–6 y(both cohorts).

	Δ z-BMI (0–6y)													
	ChildrenCohort (*n* = 632)						AdolescentCohort (*n* = 340)							
	Zero-order		Partial [1]		Partial [2]		Zero-order		Partial [1]		Partial [2]		Partial [3]	
	R	p	R	p	R	p	R	p	R	p	R	p	R	p
Aortic and peripheral blood pressure, hemodynamic and wave reflection parameters														
z-pSBP	0.20	0.003	0.28	<0.001	−0.04	0.588	0.08	0.234	0.13	0.049	0.02	0.805	0.18	0.008
z-pDBP	0.16	0.019	0.22	0.001	0.03	0.621	−0.02	0.757	0.01	0.890	−0.08	0.239	0.04	0.558
z-pPP	0.06	0.389	0.09	0.195	−0.11	0.095	0.10	0.111	0.14	0.037	0.08	0.245	0.17	0.013
z-pMBP	0.19	0.005	0.26	<0.001	0.00	0.961	0.02	0.732	0.07	0.302	−0.05	0.483	0.11	0.097
z-cSBP	0.20	0.003	0.26	<0.001	−0.04	0.529	0.02	0.765	0.16	0.014	0.05	0.483	0.20	0.003
z-cDBP	0.16	0.017	0.21	0.001	−0.04	0.567	0.00	0.977	0.11	0.083	0.06	0.380	0.12	0.074
z-cPP	0.07	0.312	0.10	0.135	0.03	0.624	0.02	0.773	0.08	0.228	0.00	0.977	0.11	0.088
z-cMBP	0.18	0.005	0.24	<0.001	−0.02	0.718	−0.04	0.556	−0.03	0.636	−0.09	0.158	0.06	0.406
z-AIx	−0.17	0.009	−0.13	0.045	0.14	0.034	0.02	0.744	0.03	0.676	0.04	0.555	0.04	0.519
z-AIx@75	−0.16	0.014	−0.17	0.009	0.19	0.005	−0.05	0.416	0.00	0.984	0.00	0.976	0.04	0.562
z-AP	−0.14	0.030	−0.09	0.161	0.12	0.056	0.02	0.735	0.04	0.590	0.05	0.439	0.05	0.485
z-Pf	0.13	0.053	0.14	0.036	−0.09	0.173	0.06	0.397	0.07	0.322	0.02	0.820	0.08	0.228
z-Pb	0.00	0.949	0.02	0.747	0.00	0.956	0.11	0.096	0.24	<0.001	0.24	<0.001	0.23	0.001
Structural arterial parameters, local and regional arterial stiffness														
z-R-CCA SD	0.24	0.016	0.29	0.003	0.05	0.639	0.09	0.146	0.12	0.066	0.00	0.968	0.17	0.011
z-R-CCA DD	0.22	0.024	0.28	0.005	0.02	0.838	0.08	0.208	0.13	0.054	0.01	0.917	0.18	0.008
z-R-CCA IMT	0.28	0.005	0.29	0.003	0.33	0.001	0.04	0.501	0.07	0.268	0.02	0.763	0.13	0.054
z-L-CCA SD	0.15	0.027	0.25	<0.001	−0.02	0.779	0.11	0.077	0.17	0.009	0.06	0.321	0.23	0.001
z-L-CCA DD	0.14	0.035	0.26	<0.001	0.03	0.623	0.10	0.121	0.20	0.002	0.09	0.189	0.26	<0.001
z-L-CCA IMT	0.14	0.043	0.20	0.002	0.13	0.044	0.12	0.069	0.17	0.007	0.13	0.048	0.24	<0.001
z-R-CFA SD	0.36	<0.001	0.33	0.002	−0.17	0.105	0.12	0.233	0.22	0.032	0.08	0.428	0.32	0.002
z-R-CFA DD	0.35	0.001	0.31	0.003	−0.18	0.094	0.11	0.281	0.18	0.075	0.05	0.645	0.28	0.007
z-R-CFA IMT	−0.25	0.296	−0.21	0.397	0.74	<0.001	0.15	0.496	0.04	0.865	−0.10	0.645	0.12	0.607
z-L-CFA SD	0.14	0.034	0.22	0.001	−0.15	0.033	0.11	0.292	0.16	0.136	0.04	0.685	0.22	0.039
z-L-CFA DD	0.12	0.071	0.19	0.004	−0.15	0.032	0.09	0.407	0.15	0.164	0.03	0.769	0.20	0.056
z-L-CFA IMT	0.17	0.250	0.12	0.413	0.36	0.013	0.01	0.967	0.36	0.073	0.26	0.218	0.30	0.149
z-R-CCA EM	0.12	0.226	0.13	0.203	0.00	0.977	−0.05	0.485	0.08	0.229	−0.01	0.850	0.12	0.080
z-L-CCA EM	0.06	0.405	0.14	0.073	0.12	0.130	0.02	0.787	0.19	0.003	0.07	0.320	0.24	<0.001
z-R-CFA EM	0.07	0.493	0.04	0.741	0.06	0.581	−0.03	0.793	−0.15	0.144	−0.14	0.184	−0.21	0.042
z-L-CFA EM	−0.06	0.407	−0.04	0.524	−0.09	0.214	−0.14	0.175	−0.08	0.436	−0.14	0.205	−0.12	0.241
z-cfPWV	−0.03	0.775	−0.04	0.625	−0.15	0.083	0.01	0.912	0.05	0.475	0.04	0.560	0.04	0.566

z: z-score. BMI: body mass index. SBP, DBP, PP, MBP: systolic, diastolic, pulse and mean pressure (p: peripheral, c: central). AIx, AIx@75: augmentation index without and with heart rate adjustment. AP: augmented pressure. Pf,Pb: forward and backward pressure components. R: Right. L: Left. CCA, CFA: common carotid and femoral artery. EM: elastic modulus. IMT: intima-media thickness. DD, SD: diastolic and systolic diameter. cfPWV: carotid-femoral pulse wave velocity. R: Pearson coefficient. *p* < 0.05 (red text) was considered significant. Partial correlations controlling for: [1] BW-for-BHz-score at birth; [2] BWH z-score at birth and z-BMI at the time of CV study; [3] BWH z-score at birth and z-BMI variation between 6 and 18 y.

Table 7. Associations between CVz-scores and z-BMI variations between 0–18y(adolescent cohort, *n* = 340).

	Δ z-BMI (0–18y)					
	Zero-Order		Partial [1]		Partial [2]	
	R	P	R	p	R	p
Aortic and peripheral blood pressure, hemodynamic and wave reflection parameters						
z-pSBP	0.14	0.021	−0.14	0.682	−0.19	0.595
z-pDBP	0.02	0.798	−0.03	0.923	0.37	0.291
z-pPP	0.14	0.016	−0.13	0.712	−0.73	0.017
z-pMBP	0.08	0.206	−0.07	0.836	0.21	0.558
z-cSBP	0.07	0.226	0.27	0.419	0.31	0.388
z-cDBP	0.03	0.613	−0.10	0.777	0.02	0.962
z-cPP	0.05	0.394	0.61	0.045	0.57	0.084
z-AIx	0.02	0.682	−0.06	0.851	0.23	0.527
z-AIx@75	0.00	0.948	−0.13	0.704	0.13	0.720
z-AP	0.02	0.741	−0.08	0.818	0.16	0.668
z-Pf	0.06	0.308	0.05	0.895	0.16	0.660
z-Pb	0.06	0.309	0.15	0.658	0.15	0.679
	Δ z-BMI (0–18y)					
	Zero-Order		Partial [1]		Partial [2]	
	R	P	R	p	R	p
Structural arterial parameters, local and regional arterial stiffness						
z-R-CCA SD	0.15	0.015	0.07	0.846	0.23	0.517
z-R-CCA DD	0.14	0.021	0.04	0.902	0.25	0.494
z-R-CCA IMT	0.03	0.604	0.15	0.667	−0.26	0.468
z-L-CCA SD	0.13	0.034	0.11	0.755	0.07	0.844

31

Table 7. *Cont.*

z-L-CCA DD	0.12	0.054	0.08	0.820	0.10	0.789
z-L-CCA IMT	0.06	0.283	−0.05	0.895	0.06	0.878
z-R-CFA SD	0.08	0.418	0.01	0.967	0.20	0.575
z-R-CFA DD	0.08	0.437	−0.08	0.806	0.18	0.615
z-R-CFA IMT	0.17	0.390	0.31	0.354	−0.16	0.656
z-L-CFA SD	0.11	0.244	−0.02	0.948	0.12	0.750
z-L-CFA DD	0.10	0.307	−0.17	0.622	0.10	0.784
z-L-CFA IMT	−0.15	0.445	0.08	0.813	0.13	0.731
z-R-CCA EM	0.02	0.788	0.38	0.254	0.33	0.359
z-L-CCA EM	0.06	0.296	0.37	0.267	0.44	0.208
z-R-CFA EM	0.02	0.821	−0.31	0.358	−0.37	0.298
z-L-CFA EM	−0.05	0.630	−0.52	0.105	−0.29	0.409
z-cfPWV	0.01	0.802	−0.29	0.387	0.32	0.367

z: z-score. BW, BH: body weight and height. BMI: body mass index. SBP, DBP, PP, MBP: systolic, diastolic, pulse and mean pressure (p: peripheral, c: central). AIx, AIx@75: augmentation index without and with heart rate adjustment. AP: augmented pressure. Pf, Pb: forward and backward pressure components. CCA, CFA: common carotid and femoral artery. EM: elastic modulus. IMT: intima-media thickness. DD, SD: diastolic and systolic diameter. cfPWV: carotid-femoral pulse wave velocity. *R*: Pearson coefficient. *p* < 0.05 (red) was considered significant. Partial correlations controlling for: [1] BW-for-BH (length) z-score at birth; [2] BW-for-BH z-score at birth and z-BMI at the time of CV study.

Table 8. Associations between CV z-scores and z-BMI variations between 6–18 y (adolescent cohort, *n* = 340).

	Δ z-BMI (6–18y)					
	Zero-Order		**Partial [1]**		**Partial [2]**	
	R	*p*	*R*	*p*	*R*	*p*
Aortic and peripheral blood pressure, hemodynamic and wave reflection parameters						
z-pSBP	0.09	0.172	−0.29	0.453	−0.24	0.566
z-pDBP	0.07	0.286	−0.31	0.419	−0.23	0.591
z-pPP	0.04	0.478	0.04	0.918	0.01	0.980
z-pMBP	0.09	0.162	−0.35	0.357	−0.27	0.521
z-cSBP	0.05	0.461	−0.22	0.565	−0.65	0.079
z-cDBP	−0.01	0.818	−0.42	0.260	−0.42	0.305
z-cPP	0.06	0.301	0.12	0.749	−0.51	0.193
z-AIx	0.03	0.602	−0.56	0.114	−0.51	0.200
z-AIx@75	0.09	0.159	−0.53	0.142	−0.45	0.264
z-AP	0.02	0.744	−0.56	0.114	−0.49	0.219
z-PF	0.02	0.707	−0.14	0.725	−0.31	0.453
z-PB	−0.08	0.211	−0.20	0.598	−0.37	0.364
Structural arterial parameters, local and regional arterial stiffness						
z-R-CCA SD	0.10	0.123	−0.55	0.123	−0.74	0.035
z-R-CCA DD	0.09	0.129	−0.38	0.308	−0.59	0.120
z-R-CCA IMT	0.12	**0.060**	0.20	0.600	−0.14	0.747
z-L-CCA SD	0.10	0.100	−0.18	0.651	−0.23	0.583
z-L-CCA DD	0.09	0.136	−0.10	0.804	−0.11	0.791
z-L-CCA IMT	0.09	0.150	−0.01	0.975	−0.33	0.418
z-R-CFA SD	0.18	**0.057**	0.14	0.722	0.13	0.754
z-R-CFA DD	0.18	**0.069**	0.10	0.795	0.30	0.475
z-R-CFA IMT	0.19	0.363	0.28	0.473	−0.34	0.415
z-L-CFA SD	0.11	0.273	−0.04	0.927	−0.14	0.748
z-L-CFA DD	0.10	0.322	−0.11	0.776	0.01	0.988
z-L-CFA IMT	−0.26	0.190	−0.28	0.470	−0.52	0.184
z-R-CCA EM	0.06	0.317	0.26	0.503	−0.20	0.631
z-L-CCA EM	0.06	0.345	0.13	0.746	−0.21	0.619
z-R-CFA EM	−0.10	0.308	0.12	0.759	0.66	0.075
z-L-CFA EM	−0.09	0.351	−0.20	0.604	0.37	0.365
z-cfPWV	−0.03	0.621	−0.63	**0.068**	−0.35	0.390

z: z-score. BW, BH: body weight and height. BMI: body mass index. SBP, DBP, PP, MBP: systolic, diastolic, pulse and mean pressure (p: peripheral, c: central). AIx, AIx@75: augmentation index without and with heart rate adjustment. AP: augmented pressure. Pf, Pb: forward and backward pressure components. CCA, CFA: common carotid and femoral artery. EM: elastic modulus. IMT: intima-media thickness. cfPWV: carotid-femoral pulse wave velocity. DD, SD: diastolic and systolic diameter. *R*: Pearson coefficient. *p* < 0.05 (red) was considered significant. Partial correlations controlling for: [1] BW-for-BH (lenght) z-score at birth; [2] BW-for-BH z-score at birth and z-BMI at the time of CV study (18 y).

Table 9. Multiple regression analysis between CVvariables (dependent) and anthropometric and CRFsvariables (independent) in children cohort (*n* = 632).

Dependent	Independent Variables	βu	SE	βs	*p*	VIF	AdjR²
Aortic and peripheral blood pressure, hemodynamic and wave reflection parameters							
z-pSBP	Constant	−0.069	0.097		0.477		0.071
	Current z-BMI	0.245	0.062	0.276	<0.001	1.00	
z-pDBP	Constant	−0.114	0.108		0.296		0.038
	Current z-BMI	0.203	0.069	0.208	0.004	1.00	
z-pPP	-	–	–	–	–	–	–
z-pMBP	Constant	−0.112	0.107		0.295		0.065
	Current z-BMI	0.247	0.068	0.255	<0.001	1.00	
z-cSBP	Constant	0.001	0.054		0.985		0.500
	z-pSBP	0.643	0.048	0.707	<0.001	1.00	
z-cDBP	Constant	−0.033	0.068		0.625		0.223
	z-pSBP	0.438	0.060	0.477	<0.001	1.00	
z-cPP	Constant	0.045	0.071		0.527		0.104
	z-pSBP	0.296	0.063	0.330	<0.001	1.00	
z-AIx	Constant	−0.059	0.072		0.414		0.099
	z-pSBP	−0.293	0.064	−0.323	<0.001	1.00	
z-AIx@75	Constant	−0.036	0.073		0.627		0.082
	z-pSBP	−0.270	0.066	−0.295	<0.001	1.00	
z-AP	Constant	−0.07	0.07		0.336		0.082
	z-pSBP	−0.23	0.06	−0.25	<0.001	1.00	
	z-BWH at birth	−0.17	0.07	−0.17	0.018	1.00	
z-Pf	Constant	0.069	0.073		0.343		0.149
	z-pSBP	0.361	0.065	0.386	<0.001	1.00	
z-Pb	Constant	−0.028	0.077		0.720		0.035
	z-pSBP	0.189	0.069	0.201	0.007	1.00	
Structural arterial parameters, local and regional arterial stiffness							
z-R-CCA SD	Constant	−0.222	0.127		**0.084**		0.173
	Current z-BMI	0.335	0.089	0.399	<0.001		
	z-pSBP	−0.205	0.091	−0.238	0.027		
z-R-CCA DD	Constant	−0.209	0.128		0.107		0.141
	Current z-BMI	0.325	0.090	0.385	0.001	1.05	
	z-pSBP	−0.200	0.092	−0.231	0.033	1.05	
z-R-CCA IMT	Constant	−0.147	0.146		0.317		0.117
	ΔBWH z-score (0–2y)	0.404	0.115	0.513	0.001	1.93	
	z-BWH at birth	0.334	0.159	0.306	0.039	1.93	
z-L-CCA SD	Constant	−0.121	0.096		0.207		0.100
	Current z-BMI	0.249	0.061	0.326	<0.001	1.00	
z-L-CCA DD	Constant	−0.071	0.086		0.414		0.099
	z-BMI	0.339	0.080	0.467	<0.001	1.22	
	Δz-BMI (0–6y) * current z-BMI	−0.050	0.023	−0.239	0.032	1.22	
z-L-CCA IMT	Constant	−0.118	0.123		0.340		0.029
	z-BMI	0.180	0.078	0.190	0.024	1.00	
z-R-CFA SD	Constant	−0.077	0.127		0.545		0.169
	Δz-BMI (0–6y)	0.347	0.090	0.411	<0.001	1.00	
z-R-CFA DD	**Constant**	−0.086	0.127		0.498		0.157
	Δz-BMI (0–6y)	0.347	0.090	0.410	<0.001	1.00	
z-R-CFA IMT	**Constant**	0.378	0.242		0.144		0.259
	Δz-BMI (0–6y)	−0.751	0.319	−0.562	0.036	1.00	

Table 9. *Cont.*

Dependent	Independent Variables	βu	SE	βs	*p*	VIF	AdjR²
z-L-CFA SD	Constant	−0.161	0.113		0.157		0.034
	Current z-BMI	0.176	0.073	0.202	0.018	1.00	
z-L-CFA DD	Constant	−0.138	0.112		0.219		0.027
	Current z-BMI	0.159	0.073	0.185	0.030	1.00	
z-L-CFA IMT	Constant	−0.046	0.175		0.796		0.222
	z-pSBP	−0.448	0.147	−0.499	0.005	1.00	
z-R-CCA EM	Constant	0.028	0.108		0.794		0.07
	z-pSBP	0.264	0.100	0.29	0.010	1.00	
z-L-CCA EM	Constant	0.068	0.085		0.429		0.03
	z-pSBP	0.160	0.075	0.18	0.034	1.00	
z-R-CFA EM	-	-	-	-	-	-	-
z-L-CFA EM	-	-	-	-	-	-	-
z-cfPWV	-	-	-	-	-	-	-

βu and βs: un- and standardized coefficients. R: Pearson coefficient. Adj R²: adjusted squared R. SE: Standard Error. VIF: variance inflation factor. z-: z-score. BMI: body mass index. SBP, DBP, PP, MBP: systolic, diastolic, pulse and mean pressure (p: peripheral, c: central). AIx, AIx@75: augmentation index without and with heart rate adjustment. AP: augmented pressure. Pf,Pb: forward and backward pressure components. CCA, CFA: common carotid and femoral artery. EM: elastic modulus. IMT: intima-media thickness. DD, SD: diastolic and systolic diameter. cfPWV: carotid-femoral pulse wave velocity. $p < 0.05$ was considered statistically significant. Variables entered in the model (forward method): z-BMI, z-BWH at birth, ΔBWH z-score 0–2y, Δ-zBMI0–6y, Sex (1: female, 0: male), z-pSBP, Hypertension (yes:1, no: 0). Interaction between growth parameters and z-BMI and z-BWH at birth were entered in the model if they showed significant association ($p < 0.005$) in the multiple linear regression. Only significant ($p < 0.05$) variables entered in the model are shown.

Explanatory variables for variations in structural parameters showed heterogeneity. At 6 y inter-individual variations in CCA SD and DD were associated with current z-BMI and z-pSBP. When considering CFA z-diameters or z-IMT levels the explanatory variables were: (a) current z-BMI (for z-left CCA IMT, CFA diameter), (b) Δz-BMI 0-6y (for z-Right CFA IMT and diameters), (c) ΔBWH z-score 0–2 y (for z-Right CCA IMT) and (d) BWH z-score at birth (for z-Right CCA IMT). Stiffness variations were not associated with anthropometric variations (Table 9). For the adolescents cohort (Table 10, Supplementary Table S14), the independent variables that remained significant in all the models ($p < 0.05$) were z-pSBP and current z-BMI (Table 10). Then, at 18 y nor BWH z-score at birth, nor the bodily changes during growth (early, intermediate, late or global), explained the CV interindividual variations (with the only exception being the interaction between current z-BMI and Δz-BMI 0-6 y for z-Right CCA IMT) (Table 10).

From the joint analysis of data from both cohorts and considering the exposure to CRFs, it can be asserted that: (1) current z-BMI was the variable mostly associated with CV characteristics; (2) the older the subject, CV properties (e.g., arterial structure) are less explained by changes in body size during the early growth phases.

Table 10. Multiple regression analysis between CVvariables (dependent) and anthropometric and CRFsvariables (independent) in adolescent cohort (*n* = 340).

Dependent Variable	Independent Variables	βu	SE	βs	*p*	VIF	Adj R²
Aortic and peripheral blood pressure, hemodynamic and wave reflection parameters							
z-pSBP	Constant	0.259	0.08		0.001		0.049
	z-BMI	0.210	0.07	0.209	0.002	1.00	
z-pDBP	-	-	-	-	-	-	-
z-pPP	Constant	0.203	0.08		0.011		0.025
	z-BMI	0.164	0.07	0.160	0.017	1.00	
z-pMBP	Constant	0.201	0.08		0.010		0.027
	z-BMI	0.164	0.07	0.165	0.014	1.00	
z-cSBP	Constant	0.024	0.05		0.663		0.424
	z-BMI	0.587	0.05	0.653	<0.001	1.00	
z-cDBP	Constant	0.039	0.07		0.591		0.178
	z-pSBP	0.422	0.06	0.426	<0.001	1.00	
z-cPP	Constant	−0.036	0.06		0.136		0.136
	z-pSBP	0.259	0.05	0.313	<0.001	1.04	
	z-BMI	0.120	0.05	0.141	0.030	1.04	
z-Aix	Constant	0.077	0.07		0.297		0.019
	z-pSBP	−0.126	0.06	−0.138	0.043	1.00	
z-Aix@75	-	-	-	-	-	-	-
z-AP	Constant	0.071	0.07		0.324		0.019
	z-pSBP	−0.139	0.06	−0.154	0.024	1.00	
z-Pf	Constant	0.015	0.07		0.829		0.098
	z-pSBP	0.270	0.06	0.313	<0.001	1.00	
z-Pb	Constant	0.070	0.07		0.334		0.060
	z-pSBP	0.219	0.06	0.245	<0.001	1.00	
Structural arterial parameters, local and regional arterial stiffness							
z-R-CCA SD	Constant	0.080	0.08		0.309		0.097
	z-BMI	0.327	0.07	0.311	<0.001	1.00	
z-R-CCA DD	Constant	−0.111	0.11		0.313		0.118
	z-BMI	0.325	0.07	0.308	<0.001	1.02	
	Sex	0.335	0.15	0.143	0.029	1.02	
z-R-CCA IMT	Constant	0.086	0.084		0.308	1.00	0.035
	Δz-BMI 0–6y * current z-BMI	0.134	0.045	0.200	0.003		
z-L-CCA SD	Constant	0.052	0.08		0.493	1.02	0.069
	z-BMI	0.255	0.06	0.263	<0.001	1.02	
z-L-CCA DD	Constant	−0.113	0.10		0.267		0.101
	z-BMI	0.252	0.06	0.267	<0.001		
	Sex	0.298	0.14	0.139	0.036	1.00	
z-L-CCA IMT	Constant	0.129	0.09		0.131		0.033
	z-BMI	0.196	0.07	0.182	0.008	1.00	
z-R-CFA SD	Constant	0.286	0.11		0.013		0.239
	z-BMI	0.343	0.10	0.331	0.001	1.03	
	Smoking	−0.609	0.22	−0.275	0.006	1.02	
	z-pSBP	−0.222	0.10	−0.223	0.025	1.01	
z-R-CFA DD	Constant	0.249	0.12		0.035		0.184
	z-BMI	0.294	0.10	0.281	0.006	1.03	
	Smoking	−0.669	0.22	−0.299	0.004	1.02	
	z-pSBP	−0.201	0.10	−0.200	0.047	1.01	
z-R-CFA IMT	Constant	0.643	0.23		0.011		0.444
	z-BMI	0.594	0.18	0.559	0.004	1.02	
	Sex	−1.067	0.39	−0.453	0.014	1.02	
z-L-CFA SD	Constant	0.140	0.12		0.229		0.066
	z-BMI	0.303	0.12	0.278	0.010	1.00	

Table 10. *Cont.*

Dependent Variable	Independent Variables	βu	SE	βs	*p*	VIF	Adj R^2
z-L-CFA DD	Constant	0.077	0.12		0.513		0.065
	z-BMI	0.304	0.12	0.275	0.011	1.00	
z-L-CFA IMT	Constant	0.175	0.231		0.456		0.557
	Hypertension	5.293	1.083	0.694	0.000	1.002	
	Dyslipemia	2.836	1.083	0.372	0.016	1.002	
z-R-CCA EM	Constant	−0.061	0.07		0.377		0.099
	z-BMI	0.213	0.06	0.233	0.001		
	z-pSBP	0.149	0.06	0.168	0.012		
z-L-CCA EM	Constant	−0.267	0.12		0.030		0.147
	z-pSBP	0.356	0.11	0.334	0.002	1.00	
z-R-CFA EM	Constant	−0.267	0.12		0.030		0.111
	z-pSBP	0.356	0.11	0.334	0.002	1.00	
z-L-CFA EM	Constant	−0.403	0.11		0.001		0.060
	z-pSBP	0.251	0.10	0.267	0.015	1.00	
z-cfPWV	Constant	−0.055	0.07		0.401		0.069
	z-pSBP	0.224	0.06	0.263	<0.001	1.00	

βu and βs: un- and standardized coefficients. R: Pearson coefficient. Adj R^2: adjusted squaredR. SE: Standard Error. VIF: variance inflation factor. z-: z-score. BMI: body mass index. SBP, DBP, PP, MBP: systolic, diastolic, pulse and mean pressure (p: peripheral, c: central). AIx, AIx@75: augmentation index without and with heart rate adjustment. AP: augmented pressure. Pf, Pb: forward and backward pressure components. CCA, CFA: common carotid and femoral artery. EM: elastic modulus. IMT: intima-media thickness. DD, SD: diastolic and systolic diameter. cfPWV: carotid-femoral pulse wave velocity. *p* < 0.05 was considered statistically significant. Variables entered in the model (forward method): z-BMI, BWH at birth, Δ-zBMI0–6y, Sex (1: female, 0: male), z-pSBP, Hypertension (1: yes, 0: no), Dislypemia (1: yes, 0: no), Smoking (1: yes, 0: no), Sedentarism (1: yes, 0: no). Interactions between growth parameters and z-BMI or z-BWH were entered in the model if they showed significant association in multiple linear regressions. Only significant (*p* < 0.05) independent variables entered in the models are shown.

4. Discussion

To our knowledge, this is the first study to describe the association of growth-related changes in body size during early, intermediate, late, or global growth with hemodynamic (central and peripheral) and arterial (structural and functional) properties in early childhood and beginning of adulthood, adjusting for characteristics at birth, at the time of the CV study and for CRFs exposure. Associations were assessed considering three interrelated comparative analysis: (1) strength and (2) independence of the associations and (3) explanatory power of anthropometric parameters and factors associated with CV risk. Our main findings were:

- First, growth-related body size changes (0–2 and 0–6 y) were associated with interindividual variations (z-score) in CV properties at 6 y. Conversely, CV z-scores variables at 18 y were not associated with body size changes (0–6, 6–18 or 0–18 y) (Tables 2 and 3). Thus, as the subject's age increases, the association between CV properties and prior body size changes (i.e., during childhood) decreases (Table 4).
- Second, the strength of association between growth-related body changes and CV properties at 6 y was: (a) equal or greater than that observed for body size at birth and (b) lower than the obtained for current z-BMI (at 6 y). Most of the associations between ΔBWH z-score 0–2 y or Δz-BMI 0–6 y and the CV properties at 6 y were independent of the BWH z-score at birth (Tables 5 and 6). Then, in 6 y children the "hierarchical order" among explanatory variables for CV variations would be: current z-BMI > ΔBWH z-score 0–2 y or Δz-BMI 0–6 y> BWH z-score at birth (Table 2). On the contrary, only current z-BMI showed significant association with CV properties at 18 y (Table 3). In summary, while current z-BMI showed the strongest association, body size at birth showed almost no association with CV properties, regardless of subjects' age at the time of the CV study (Tables 2 and 3).
- Third, in general terms, current z-BMI was the anthropometric parameter with the greatest explanatory capacity for CV variations observed at 6 y. Though, variations in some CV parameters

were mainly explained by growth-related body changes and/or by their interaction with current z-BMI (Tables S4 and S6). Similar results were observed when the associations were analyzed considering the exposure to CRFs (e.g., hypertension, dyslipidemia) (Table 9). In turn, current z-BMI was the anthropometric variable with the greatest explanatory capacity for CV conditions and variations at 18 y.In summary, body size changes during childhood and/or adolescence contributed to explain arterial variations through the interaction with current z-BMI or BWH z-score at birth (Tables S8, S10 and S12). Among factors associated with CV risk, z-BMI and/or z-pSBP were the main explanatory variables for CV z-scores (Table 10).

The explanatory capacity of growth-related body changes was reduced or lost with, as the age at which the CV system was evaluated increased. In this regard, at least two issues must be analyzed. On the one hand, the impact (association) of anthropometric changes on the CV properties evaluated at a given age, would vary, depending on the period of "body change or gain" considered (e.g., 0–2 y vs. 0–6 y). On the other hand, the association between CV properties and the anthropometric changes observed in a given period (e.g., 0–6 y) could depend on the age at which the CV system is evaluated (e.g., 6 vs. 18 y, like in this work). Studies suggested that BW gain patterns in very early infancy (e.g., 0–6 postnatal mos.) [22–24] would be particularly important as determinants of future pBP levels, while other studies showed that BW gain during childhood would be a stronger predictor of pBP [25,26]. The exact "timing of the BW gain" associated with middle or long-term CV risk is still debated, highlighting the need for additional research to clarify and/or reconcile mixed findings. In this work, in general terms we did not find differences in the strength of association when comparing 0–2 vs. 0–6 y data, but some CV characteristics assessed at 6 y showed greater association with 0–6 y anthropometric changes. Evelein et al. (2013) reported that postnatal BW for length gain (0-3 mos.) was associated with carotid IMT (but not stiffness) in children (5 y) [21]. However, when data about growth in later infancy (3–6, 6–9 and 9–12 mos.) were considered, no associations with arterial properties were found [21]. Skilton et al. (2013) reported that BW gain, BH-adjusted-BW gain and ΔBWH z-score 0-18 mos. were positively associated with carotid IMT assessed at 8 y [27]. Unfortunately, the impact of changes in different periods was not analyzed. Linhares et al. (2015) found that the "adverse" long-term effect of accelerated growth in infancy varied depending on the time of growth acceleration. Particularly, carotid IMT at ~30 y was associated with 2–4 y BW-gain, rather than with early BW gain [7]. Additionally, Vianna et al. (2016), found that the relative BW-gain between 2 and 4 y was associated with increased aortic stiffness (evaluated by cfPWV) at ~30 y, whereas birth weight, BW-gain within the first 2 years of life (0–2 y) and linear growth (length/height gain) in childhood were not associated with cfPWV [28]. Pais et al. (2016) assessed PWV in children (8–9 y) and analyzed data considering and categorizing growth trajectories. The highest arterial stiffness levels were observed in groups with accelerated body growth during childhood, with adequate early growth pattern [29].

The dependence on the age at the time of CV study ascribed to the association between an anthropometric parameter and CV properties has been previously described, mainly for birth weight. About this, body size at birth has been associated with pBP levels, andit was reported that the relation becomes progressively stronger with increasing age, being hypothesized that the initiating process occurs in uterus and amplifies throughout life [11,30,31], satisfying theories that seek to explain the detriment of the CV system related to low birth weight and/or catch-up growth [32]. It was even postulated that interactions between increased arterial stiffness, increased pPP, stretching of vascular smooth muscles and synthesis of collagen may contribute to the amplification phenomenon through a feedback loop [33]. By contrast, Lule et al. analyzed data from studies that measured pBP at different ages and did not find an age-related increase in the strength of the association between birth weight and pBP [6]. Furthermore, the relationship between birth weight and later pBP varied depending on the age of the participants: neonates showed consistent positive association; mainly negative associations were seen in children, and studies in adolescents showed inconsistent results [6]. Then, as age increases, the positive association observed in neonates could become negative, non-existent or even positive, which is in agreement with our findings. This could be explained, at least in theory by the fact that as age increases the exposure-time to already present factors capable of impacting on the CV system also increases. As age increases, subjects could become exposed to factors (i.e., CRFs) capable of modifyingCV properties. Then, the association between anthropometricchanges and CVproperties could be modified by exposure to co-factors.

As mentioned in 6 y children the "hierarchical order" among explanatory variables for CV variations would be: current z-BMI >ΔBWH z-score 0–2 y or Δz-BMI 0–6 y> BWH z-score at birth (Table 2). Conversely, only current z-BMI showed significant association with arterial properties at 18 y (Table 3). Birth weight showed almost no association with CV properties, disregard of the subjects' age at the time of the CV study (Tables 2 and 3), and most of the associations between ΔBWH z-score 0–2 y or Δz-BMI 0–6 y and CV characteristics at 6 ywere independent of birth conditions (Tables 5 and 6). Then, the association between body-size changes during infancy or childhood and the CV system at 6 y, would not depend on having been born with low, normal or elevated BWH. When current z-BMI was considered some associations between bodily changes in childhood and CV properties at 6 y were no longer significant. In adolescents, the associations between body changes and CV variables were always dependent on z-BMI at the time of CV study (Tables 6–8).

The dependence (or independence) of the association between CV parameters and growth–related anthropometric changes on bodysize at birth and/or on current z-BMI has been previously assessed, with dissimilar findings. A positive association was observed between BW gain or adiposity accumulation during childhood and later pBP levels [23,34–37]. However, the extent to which birth size modifies the associations between postnatal growth and future pBP levels and/or arterial properties remains unclear. Belfort et al. (2007) found that infants who were thinner at birth were more susceptible to adverse effects on pBP at 3 y of accelerated BWH gain within the first 6 postnatal mos. [22]. Whether the finding is extensive to mid-childhood when BP is highly correlated with adult BP [38] is to be clarified. Leunissen et al. (2012) showed that regardless of birth-size, adiposity accumulation during childhood is a risk factor for later (~20 y) development of high BP levels [37]. Accordingly, Kelishadi's review (2014) concludes that early growth, rather than birth weight, would be important as a determinant of later BP levels [32]. Supporting a BMI-independent association between body size changes and CV properties, Thiering et al. studied children ($n = 1127$, age≤10 y) and reported that higher BW peak (velocity) in infancy was associated with an increase in pSBP and pDBP after confounders adjustment [39]. In contrast, it has been proposed that the association between BMI at adiposity peak and BP at 6 y would be mediated by current BMI [40]. Marinkovic et al. (2017) observed that infant peak BW velocity and BMI at adiposity peak associationwith childhood pSBP and pDBP (at 6 y), which could be explained by current BMI [12].

Our results support the proposal that the association between anthropometric parameters and pBP depends on current BMI, at the same time as they provide original information showing that unlike what was described for pBP, the association between growth-related body size changes (0–2 y) and cBP at 6 y would not depend on current z-BMI. This is further supported by the fact that reflection parameters, which are main determinants of the differences between cBPand pBP, also showed associations not explained by current BMI (Tables 5 and 6). It is to note that compared to pBP, the cBP would be of greater value in terms of association with CVchanges and risk prediction [41].

As stated above, the association between growth-related body-size changes and arterial thickness has been previously described [21,27,42]. Our results provide additional information, showing that at 6 y, the association between body size gain and thickness is independent of body size at birth and current z-BMI at 6 y, and that it is statistical significant for both carotid (elastic) and femoral (muscular) arteries. In turn, Evelein et al. (2013) described interaction between birth size and postnatal weight for length by analyzing the impact on arterial stiffness (i.e., distensibility and arterial elastic modulus). The thinner the children were at birth, the lower the distensibility (greater the elastic modulus) with increasing weight for length gain [21]. Then, the impact of birth-size and or growth-related changes would vary depending on the CV properties considered.

Finally, as mentioned, current z-BMI was the anthropometric parameter with the greatest explanatory capacity (power) for the CV variations observed at 6 and 18 y. However, interindividual variations in some hemodynamic and arterial parameters at 6 and 18 y were mainly explained by growth-related body changes and/or by their interaction with current z-BMI (Tables S4 and S6 for children; Tables S8, S10 and S12 for adolescents). Similar results were observed when the associations were analyzed taking into account the exposure to CRFs (Tables 9 and 10). In children, body change during growth, independently or by means of an interaction with current z-BMI, allowed to explain to a greater extent some CV characteristics (i.e., arterial thicknesses and diameters). In other words, disregard of birth size, exposure to CRFs and/or z-pBP, arterial wall thickness and/or diameters at 6 y could be explained by body growth between 0–2 or 0–6 y. Thus, although CV properties at 6 y would be associated with current z-BMI, knowing the history of BW gain could contribute to a better understanding of the CV characteristics of a specific child. Two children with similar z-BMI, could present CV differences associated with their "history" of body size changes (e.g., between 0–2 or 0–6y). Furthermore, for variables such as wall thickness in children, the history of weight gain would have greater explanatory capacity than current z-BMI or factors with recognized impact on the CV system (e.g., CRFs). In adolescents, the history of BW gain would not be a primary explanatory variable for CV variables (i.e., for IMT), but due to variables interactions it could contribute or complement data obtained from current z-BMI and/or BP.

5. Strengths and Limitations

This work has several strengths that should be considered. First, the population-based prospective cohort design, including a large number of subjects studied from early life. Repeated measures during growth-period enabled us to study the impact of growth profiles or patterns on CV properties, assessed at two specific times: early childhood (6 y) and onset of adulthood (18 y). Second, we used our own specific "reference populations" to define CV z-scores (Supplementary Tables S1 and S2). Third, many potential confounders were considered in order to isolate the effect of BW gain in the statistical models. Fourth, taking into account that the impact of body change on the CV system may depend on the period in which it occurs, we studied different periods of body gain (0–2, 0–6, 0–18, 6–18 y). Fifth, the relationship between BW gain and adult pBP is one of the most studied, based on the "fetal origin" hypothesis, but pBP is a particular variable and does not inform about central hemodynamic conditions, or about structural and/or functional arterial changes (e.g., associated with early vascular aging or atherosclerosis development). Thus, we designed an integral approach in which multiple CV parameters (e.g., pBP, cBP, arterial diameters and thicknesses, local and regional stiffness) and different arterial pathways (i.e., elastic and muscular) were evaluated. Sixth, unlike most works that analyzed the associations between body changes and the CV system considering a single age, we studied children and young adults. Up to now, most studies included premature, small for gestational age, obese and/or hypertensive subjects and data about the CV impact of growth-related body changes in healthy pediatric and/or adolescent populations were scarce. In this work, healthy children and adolescents were studied.

Some limitations should be considered. First, we did not have information about blood biomarkers measured by our technicians. Therefore data about some conditions (i.e., existence of dyslipidemia) was obtained from reference physicians, registers and/or self-reports. Second, although we adjusted for several potential confounders, residual confounding factors may persist, as in any observational study. Third, in this work we chose to use change in BWH z-score or z-BMI between two time points as growth-indicators. This approach is a simple practical (clinical) method for quantifying a "change"; although more detailed growth patterns could be derived from longitudinally collected anthropometric measures in both cohorts. Fourth, we did not perform an analysis discriminating by sex; despite we are aware of data suggesting that the impact of childhood growth on the CV system may differ between boys and girls [12]. Fifth, we included subjects born at term and preterm, but as most of them belonged to the first condition (98% and 92% in children and adolescent cohorts, respectively) the results should be assigned to term-born subjects. Sixth, comparative analysis of the associations between anthropometric data and CV (hemodynamic and/or arterial) variables measured at 6 and 18 y was done considering two different cohorts, instead of a single cohort followed for more than 20 years. Although obtaining similar data for different cohorts could be considered as strength of the work, as a limiting factor it should be noted that for some variables data were not obtained in both cohorts and some aspects of the associations could only be evaluated in one of them. Finally, we did not analyze growth considering body composition (e.g., fat mass) and its changes as was previously done [43].

6. Conclusions

Body-size changes in infancy (0–2 y) and childhood (0–6 y) showed similar strength of association with respect to CV properties assessed at 6 y. Conversely, changes between 0–6, 6-18 or 0–18 y were not associated with CV parameters evaluated at 18 y.

The association between CV characteristics at 6 yand body-size changes during growth showed: (a) equal or greater strength than the observed for body-size at birth, and (b) lower strength with respect to that obtained when considering current z-BMI at 6 y. In 6 y children variables capable of explaining CV variations showed a "hierarchical order". Conversely, only z-BMI at 18 y showed significant associations with arterial z-scores at 18 y. Body size at birth showed almost no association with arterial characteristics at 6 or 18 y. The associations between ΔBWH z-score 0–2 y or Δz-BMI 0–6 y and CV properties at 6 y were mostly independent of body-size at birth. When current z-BMI was taken into account some associations between body changes in childhood and CV properties at 6 y were no longer significant. In adolescents, the associations between growth-related body changes and CV properties were dependent on z-BMI at the time of CVstudy.

Current z-BMI was the anthropometric parameter with the greatest capacity to explain the variations in CV properties at 6 y. However, interindividual variations in some hemodynamic and arterial parameters were mainly explained by growth-related anthropometric changes and/or by their interaction with current z-BMI. Similar findings were observed when the associations were analyzed taking into account the exposure to factors associated with CV risk. Current z-BMI at 18 y was the anthropometric variable with the greatest capacity to explain CV variations at 18 y. Body-size changes during childhood and/or adolescence contributed to explain arterial variations through the interaction with current z-BMI or BWH z-score at birth.

Supplementary Materials: The following are available online at http://www.mdpi.com/2308-3425/6/3/33/s1. Table S1. Clinical, anthropometric hemodynamic, structural and stiffness parameters forchildren and adolescent reference subgroups; Table S2. Hemodynamic, structural and stiffness parameters z-score, forchildren and adolescent Cohorts; Table S3. Multiple linear regression analysis between CVparameters z-scores (dependent variables) and anthropometric parameters (independent variables), children cohort (*n* = 632); Table S4. Multiple linear regression analysis between CV parameters z-scores (dependent variables) and anthropometric parameters (independent variables), children cohort (*n* = 632); Table S5. Multiple linear regression analysis between CV parameters z-scores (dependent variables) and anthropometric parameters (independent variables), children cohort (*n* = 632); Table S6. Multiple linear regression analysis between CV parameters z-scores (dependent variables) and anthropometric parameters (independent variables), children cohort (*n* = 632); Table S7. Multiple linear regression analysis between CV parameters z-scores (dependent variables) and anthropometric parameters (independent variables), adolescent cohort (*n* = 340); Table S8. Multiple linear regression analysis between CV parameters z-scores (dependent variables) and anthropometric parameters (independent variables), adolescent cohort (*n* = 340); Table S9. Multiple linear regression analysis between CV parameters z-scores (dependent variables) and anthropometric parameters (independent variables), adolescent cohort (*n* = 340); Table S10. Multiple linear regression analysis between CV parameters z-scores (dependent variables) and anthropometric parameters (independent variables), adolescent cohort (*n* = 340); Table S11. Multiple linear regression analysis between CV parameters z-scores (dependent variables) and anthropometricparameters (independent variables), adolescent cohort (*n* = 340); Table S12. Multiple linear regression analysis between CV parameters z-scores (dependent variables) and anthropometric parameters (independent variables), adolescent cohort (*n* = 340); Table S13. Multiple linear regression analysis between CV parameters z-scores (dependent variables) and anthropometric parameters and CVRFs (independent variables), children cohort (*n* = 632) (Enter Method); Table S14. Multiple linear regression analysis between CV parameters z-scores (dependent variables) and anthropometric parameters and CVRFs (independent variables), adolescent cohort (*n* = 340) (Enter Method)

J. Cardiovasc. Dev. Dis. **2019**, *6*, 33

Author Contributions: Conceptualization, D.B. and Y.Z.; Formal analysis, J.M.C., D.B. and Y.Z.; Funding acquisition, D.B. and Y.Z.; Investigation, D.B. and Y.Z.; Methodology, J.M.C., V.G.-E., A.Z., M.M., C.S., D.B. and Y.Z.; Project administration, D.B. and Y.Z.; Visualization, J.M.C., D.B. and Y.Z.; Writing–original draft, J.M.C., D.B. and Y.Z.; Writing–review and editing, J.M.C., V.G.-E., A.Z., M.M., C.S., P.C., D.B. and Y.Z.

Funding: This research was funded by Agencia Nacional de Investigación e Innovación (ANII), Ministry for Social Development (MIDES), United Nations Children's Fund (UNICEF), grant number/code: FSPI_X_2015_1_108484, PRSCT-008-020; and extrabudgetary funds provided by CUiiDARTE.

Acknowledgments: We thank the children, adolescents and their families for their participation in the study. The authors thank the technical staff from CUiiDARTE and IECON (Lic. Cecilia Toledo and LucíaNuñez). ELBU Study (IECON; http://fcea.edu.uy/estudio-del-bienestar-multidimensional-en-uruguay.html) is directed by Martín Leites, Gonzalo Salas and Andrea Vigorito.

Conflicts of Interest: The authors declare no conflict of interest. The funders had no role in the design of the study; in the collection, analyses, or interpretation of data; in the writing of the manuscript, or in the decision to publish the results.

Abbreviations

AIx	central (aortic) augmentation index
AIx@75	AIx adjusted to a 75 beats/min heart rate
AP	central (aortic) augmented pressure
BH	body height
BMI	body mass index
BW	body weight
BWH	body weight for body height
cBP	central (aortic) blood pressure
CCA	common carotid artery
CFA	common femoral artery
cfPWV	carotid-femoral pulse wave velocity
CRFs	cardiovascular risk factors
CV	cardiovascular
CVD	cardiovascular disease
DD	diastolic arterial diameter
EM	pressure-strain arterial elastic modulus
HBP	high blood pressure levels
HR	heart rate
IMT	intima-media thickness
LBW	low birth weight
MLR	multiple linear regression models
mos.	Months
MV	mean value
Pb	amplitude of the cBP backward component
pBP	peripheral (brachial) blood pressure
pDBP	peripheral (brachial) diastolic blood pressure
Pf	amplitude of the cBP forward component
pMBP	peripheral (brachial) mean blood pressure
pPP	peripheral (brachial) pulse pressure
pSBP	peripheral (brachial) systolic blood pressure
PWA	pulse wave analysis
SD	systolic arterial diameter
STD	standard deviation
VIF	variance inflation factor
y	years old
z	z-score

References

1. Ayer, J.G.; Harmer, J.A.; Nakhla, S.; Xuan, W.; Ng, M.K.; Raitakari, O.T.; Marks, G.B.; Celermajer, D.S. HDL-cholesterol, blood pressure, and asymmetric dimethylarginine are significantly associated with arterial wall thickness in children. *Arterioscler. Thromb. Vasc. Biol.* **2009**, *29*, 943–949. [CrossRef] [PubMed]
2. Umer, A.; Kelley, G.A.; Cottrell, L.E.; Giacobbi, P., Jr.; Innes, K.E.; Lilly, C.L. Childhood obesity and adult cardiovascular disease risk factors: A systematic review with meta-analysis. *BMC Public Health* **2017**, *17*, 683. [CrossRef] [PubMed]
3. Weihrauch-Blüher, S.; Schwarz, P.; Klusmann, J.H. Childhood obesity: Increased risk for cardiometabolic disease and cancer in adulthood. *Metabolism* **2019**, *92*, 147–152. [CrossRef] [PubMed]
4. Huxley, R.; Neil, A.; Collins, R. Unravelling the fetal origins hypothesis: Is there really an inverse association between birthweight and subsequent blood pressure? *Lancet* **2002**, *360*, 659–665. [CrossRef]
5. Leunissen, R.W.; Kerkhof, G.F.; Stijnen, T.; Hokken-Koelega, A. Timing and tempo of first-year rapid growth in relation to cardiovascular and metabolic risk profile in early adulthood. *JAMA* **2009**, *301*, 2234–2242. [CrossRef] [PubMed]
6. Lule, S.A.; Elliott, A.M.; Smeeth, L.; Webb, E.L. Is birth weight associated with blood pressure among African children and adolescents? A systematic review. *J. Dev. Orig. Health Dis.* **2018**, *9*, 270–280. [CrossRef] [PubMed]
7. da Silva Linhares, R.; Gigante, D.P.; de Barros, F.C.; Horta, B.L. Carotid intima-media thickness at age 30, birth weight, accelerated growth during infancy and breastfeeding: A birth cohort study in Southern Brazil. *PLoS ONE* **2015**, *10*, e0115166.
8. Adair, L.S.; Fall, C.H.D.; Osmond, C.; Stein, A.D.; Martorell, R.; Ramirez-Zea, M.; Sachdev, H.S.; Dahly, D.L.; Bas, I.; Norris, S.A.; et al. Associations of linear growth and relative weight gain during early life with adult health and human capital in countries of low and middle income: Findings from five birth cohort studies. *Lancet* **2013**, *382*, 525–534. [CrossRef]
9. Ong, K.K.; Ahmed, M.L.; Emmett, P.M.; Preece, M.A.; Dunger, D.B. Association between postnatal catch-up growth and obesity in childhood: Prospective cohort study. *BMJ* **2000**, *320*, 967–971. [CrossRef]
10. Jansen, M.A.C.; Uiterwaal, C.S.P.M.; van der Ent, C.K.; Grobbee, D.E.; Dalmeijer, G.W. Excess early postnatal weight gain and blood pressure in healthy young children. *J. Dev. Orig. Health Dis.* **2019**, *30*, 1–7. [CrossRef]
11. Law, C.M.; de Swiet, M.; Osmond, C.; Fayers, P.M.; Barker, D.J.; Cruddas, A.M.; Fall, C.H. Initiation of hypertension in utero and its amplification throughout life. *BMJ* **1993**, *306*, 24–27. [CrossRef] [PubMed]
12. Marinkovic, T.; Toemen, L.; Kruithof, C.J.; Reiss, I.; van Osch-Gevers, L.; Hofman, A.; Franco, O.H.; Jaddoe, V.W.V. Early infant growth velocity patterns and cardiovascular and metabolic outcomes in childhood. *J. Pediatr.* **2017**, *186*, 57–63. [CrossRef] [PubMed]
13. Garcia-Espinosa, V.; Bia, D.; Castro, J.; Zinoveev, A.; Marin, M.; Giachetto, G.; Chiesa, P.; Zócalo, Y. Peripheral and central aortic pressure, wave-derived reflection parameters, local and regional arterial stiffness and structural parameters in children and adolescents: Impact of body mass index variations. *High Blood Press. Cardiovasc. Prev.* **2018**, *25*, 267–280. [CrossRef] [PubMed]
14. Zócalo, Y.; Ungerfeld, R.; Pérez-Clariget, R.; Bia, D. Maternal nutritional restriction during gestation impacts differently on offspring muscular and elastic arteries and is associated with increased carotid resistance and ventricular afterload in maturity. *J. Dev. Orig. Health Dis.* **2019**, 1–11. [CrossRef] [PubMed]
15. Zócalo, Y.; Curcio, S.; García-Espinosa, V.; Chiesa, P.; Giachetto, G.; Bia, D. Comparative analysis of arterial parameters variations associated with inter-individual variations in peripheral and aortic blood pressure: Cross-sectional study in healthy subjects aged 2-84 years. *High Blood Press. Cardiovasc. Prev.* **2017**, *24*, 437–451. [CrossRef] [PubMed]
16. Zócalo, Y.; Castro, J.M.; Garcia-Espinosa, V.; Curcio, S.; Chiesa, P.; Giachetto, G.; Cabrera-Fischer, E.I.; Bia, D. Forward and backward aortic components and reflection indexes in children and adolescents: Determinants and role in high pressure states. *Curr. Hypertens. Rev.* **2018**, *14*, 137–153. [CrossRef] [PubMed]
17. Amarante, V.; Arim, R.; Severi, C.; Vigorito, A.; Aldabe, I.; de Melo, G.; Rodríguez, A.; Salas, G. *El Estadonutricional de los NiñOs/as y las Políticasalimentarías*; Programa Naciones Unidas para e Desarrollo (PNUD)-UNICEF: Montevideo, Uruguay, 2007.

18. Lurbe, E.; Agabiti-Rosei, E.; Cruickshank, J.K.; Dominiczak, A.; Erdine, S.; Hirth, A.; Invitti, C.; Litwin, M.; Mancia, G.; Pall, D.; et al. 2016 European Society of Hypertension guidelines for the management of high blood pressure in children and adolescents. *J. Hypertens.* **2016**, *34*, 1887–1920. [CrossRef] [PubMed]
19. García-Espinosa, V.; Curcio, S.; Marotta, M.; Castro, J.M.; Arana, M.; Peluso, G.; Chiesa, P.; Giachetto, G.; Bia, D.; Zócalo, Y. Changes in central aortic pressure levels, wave components and determinants associated with high peripheral blood pressure states in childhood: Analysis of hypertensive phenotype. *Pediatr. Cardiol.* **2016**, *37*, 1340–1350. [CrossRef] [PubMed]
20. Diedenhofen, B.; Musch, J. Cocor: A comprehensive solution for the statistical comparison of correlations. *PLoS ONE* **2015**, *10*, e0121945. [CrossRef] [PubMed]
21. Evelein, A.M.; Visseren, F.L.; van der Ent, C.K.; Grobbee, D.E.; Uiterwaal, C.S. Excess early postnatal weight gain leads to thicker and stiffer arteries in young children. *J. Clin. Endocrinol. Metab.* **2013**, *98*, 794–801. [CrossRef] [PubMed]
22. Belfort, M.B.; Rifas-Shiman, S.L.; Rich-Edwards, J.; Kleinman, K.P.; Gillman, M.W. Size at birth, infant growth, and blood pressure at three years of age. *J. Pediatr.* **2007**, *151*, 670–674. [CrossRef] [PubMed]
23. Ben-Shlomo, Y.; McCarthy, A.; Hughes, R.; Tilling, K.; Davies, D.; Smith, G.D. Immediate postnatal growth is associated with blood pressure in young adulthood: The Barry Caerphilly Growth Study. *Hypertension* **2008**, *52*, 638–644. [CrossRef] [PubMed]
24. Adair, L.S.; Martorell, R.; Stein, A.D.; Hallal, P.C.; Sachdev, H.S.; Prabhakaran, D.; Wills, A.K.; Norris, S.A.; Dahly, D.L.; Lee, N.R.; et al. Size at birth, weight gain in infancy and childhood, and adult blood pressure in 5 low- and middle-income-country cohorts: When does weight gain matter? *Am. J. Clin. Nutr.* **2009**, *89*, 1383–1392. [CrossRef] [PubMed]
25. Jones, A.; Charakida, M.; Falaschetti, E.; Hingorani, A.D.; Finer, N.; Masi, S.; Donald, A.E.; Lawlor, D.A.; Smith, G.D.; Deanfield, J.E. Adipose height growth through childhood blood pressure status in a large prospective cohort, s.t.u.d.y. *Hypertension* **2012**, *59*, 919–925. [CrossRef] [PubMed]
26. Tilling, K.; Davies, N.; Windmeijer, F.; Kramer, M.S.; Bogdanovich, N.; Matush, L.; Patel, R.; Smith, G.D.; Ben-Shlomo, Y.; Martin, R.M. Is infant weight associated with childhood blood pressure? Analysis of the promotion of breastfeeding intervention trial (probit) cohort. *Int. J. Epidemiol.* **2011**, *40*, 1227–1237. [CrossRef] [PubMed]
27. Skilton, M.R.; Marks, G.B.; Ayer, J.G.; Garden, F.L.; Garnett, S.P.; Harmer, J.A.; Leeder, S.R.; Toelle, B.G.; Webb, K.; Baur, L.A.; et al. Weight gain in infancy and vascular risk factors in later childhood. *Pediatrics* **2013**, *131*, 1821–1828. [CrossRef] [PubMed]
28. Vianna, C.A.; Horta, B.L.; Gigante, D.P.; de Barros, F.C. Pulse wave velocity at early adulthood: Breastfeeding and nutrition during pregnancy and childhood. *PLoS ONE* **2016**, *11*, e0152501. [CrossRef] [PubMed]
29. Pais, C.; Correia-Costa, L.; Moura, C.; Mota, C.; Severo, M.; Guerra, A.; Areias, J.C.; Schaefer, F.; CaldasAfonso, A.; Barros, H.; et al. Accelerated growth during childhood is associated with increased arterial stiffness in prepubertal children. *Int. J. Cardiol.* **2016**, *204*, 83–85. [CrossRef]
30. Huxley, R.R.; Shiell, A.W.; Law, C.M. The role of size at birth and postnatal catch-up growth in determining systolic blood pressure: A systematic review of the literature. *J. Hypertens.* **2000**, *18*, 815–831. [CrossRef]
31. Law, C.M.; Shiell, A.W. Is blood pressure inversely related to birth weight? The strength of evidence from a systematic review of the literature. *J. Hypertens.* **1996**, *14*, 935–941. [CrossRef]
32. Kelishadi, R.; Haghdoost, A.A.; Jamshidi, F.; Aliramezany, M.; Moosazadeh, M. Low birthweight or rapid catch-up growth: Which is more associated with cardiovascular disease and its risk factors in later life? A systematic review and cryptanalysis. *Paediatr. Int. Child Health* **2015**, *35*, 110–123. [CrossRef] [PubMed]
33. Martyn, C.N.; Greenwald, S.E. Impaired synthesis of elastin in walls of aorta and large conduit arteries during early development as an initiating event in pathogenesis of systemic hypertension. *Lancet* **1997**, *350*, 953–955. [CrossRef]
34. Uiterwaal, C.S.; Anthony, S.; Launer, L.J.; Witteman, J.C.; Trouwborst, A.M.; Hofman, A.; Grobbee, D.E. Birth weight, growth, and blood pressure: An annual follow-up study of children aged 5 through 21 years. *Hypertension* **1997**, *30*, 267–271. [CrossRef] [PubMed]
35. Adair, L.S.; Cole, T.J. Rapid child growth raises blood pressure in adolescent boys who were thin at birth. *Hypertension* **2003**, *41*, 451–456. [CrossRef] [PubMed]

36. Nishina, M.; Kikuchi, T.; Yamazaki, H.; Kameda, K.; Hiura, M.; Uchiyama, M. Relationship among systolic blood pressure, serum insulin and leptin, and visceral fat accumulation in obese children. *Hypertens. Res.* **2003**, *26*, 281–288. [CrossRef] [PubMed]
37. Leunissen, R.W.; Kerkhof, G.F.; Stijnen, T.; Hokken-Koelega, A.C. Effect of birth size and catch-up growth on adult blood pressure and carotid intima-media thickness. *Horm. Res. Paediatr.* **2012**, *77*, 394–401. [CrossRef] [PubMed]
38. Chen, X.; Wang, Y. Tracking of blood pressure from childhood to adulthood: A systematic review and meta-regression analysis. *Circulation* **2008**, *117*, 3171–3180. [CrossRef] [PubMed]
39. Thiering, E.; Bruske, I.; Kratzsch, J.; Hoffmann, B.; Herbarth, O.; von Berg, A.; Schaaf, B.; Wichmann, H.E.; Heinrich, J.; LISAplus Study Group. Peak growth velocity in infancy is positively associated with blood pressure in school-aged children. *J. Hypertens.* **2012**, *30*, 1114–1121. [CrossRef]
40. Hof, M.H.; Vrijkotte, T.G.; de Hoog, M.L.; van Eijsden, M.; Zwinderman, A.H. Association between infancy BMI peak and body composition and blood pressure at age 5–6 years. *PLoS ONE* **2013**, *8*, e80517. [CrossRef]
41. Peluso, G.; García-Espinosa, V.; Curcio, S.; Marota, M.; Castro, J.; Chiesa, P.; Giachetto, G.; Bia, D.; Zócalo, Y. High central aortic rather than brachial blood pressure is associated with carotid wall remodeling and increased arterial stiffness in childhood. *High Blood Press. Cardiovasc. Prev.* **2017**, *24*, 49–60. [CrossRef]
42. Skilton, M.R.; Sullivan, T.R.; Ayer, J.G.; Garden, F.L.; Harmer, J.A.; Leeder, S.R.; Toelle, B.G.; Webb, K.; Marks, G.B.; Celermajer, D.S. Weight gain in infancy is associated with carotid extra-medial thickness in later childhood. *Atherosclerosis* **2014**, *233*, 370–374. [CrossRef] [PubMed]
43. McCloskey, K.; Burgner, D.; Carlin, J.B.; Skilton, M.R.; Cheung, M.; Dwyer, T.; Vuillermin, P.; Ponsonby, A.L.; BIS Investigator Group. Infant adiposity at birth and early postnatal weight gain predict increased aortic intima-media thickness at 6 weeks of age: A population-derived cohort study. *Clin. Sci. (Lond.)* **2016**, *130*, 443–450. [CrossRef] [PubMed]

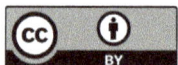

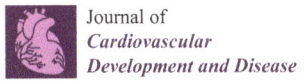

Article

Dietary Adherence of Saudi Males to the Saudi Dietary Guidelines and Its Relation to Cardiovascular Diseases: A Preliminary Cross-Sectional Study

Areej Ali Alkhaldy [1,*], Reem Saleh Alamri [1], Rozana Khalid Magadmi [1], Nrvana Yasser Elshini [1], Rania Abd El Hamid Hussein [1,2] and Kamal Waheeb Alghalayini [3]

[1] Clinical Nutrition Department, Faculty of Applied Medical Sciences, King Abdulaziz University, P.O. Box 80215, Jeddah 21589, Saudi Arabia; reemsalamri@gmail.com (R.S.A.); rozana-magadmi@hotmail.com (R.K.M.); nrvanaalshini@gmail.com (N.Y.E.); rahussein2002@yahoo.com (R.A.E.H.H.)
[2] Internal Medicine Department, Gamal Abd El Nasser Hospital, Health Insurance Authority, Alexandria 21516, Egypt
[3] Department of Medicine, Faculty of Medicine, King Abdulaziz University, P.O. Box 80215, Jeddah 21589, Saudi Arabia; kalghalayini@kau.edu.sa
* Correspondence: aalkhaldy@kau.edu.sa; Tel.: +966-12-6400000 (ext. 24215)

Received: 2 February 2019; Accepted: 2 April 2019; Published: 4 April 2019

Abstract: Cardiovascular disease (CVD) is a major public health problem in Saudi Arabia. Dietary intake plays a major role in CVD incidence; however, the dietary intake status in Saudi nationals with CVD is unknown. We aimed to investigate whether the dietary patterns of Saudi males, using the Saudi dietary guidelines adherence score, in parallel with the measurement of a selective number of cardiovascular disease-related biomarkers, are contributing factors to CVD risk. Demographics, dietary adherence score, and blood biomarker levels were collected for 40 CVD patients and forty non-CVD patients. Fasting blood glucose ($p = 0.006$) and high-density lipoprotein levels ($p = 0.03$) were significantly higher in CVD patients. The adherence score to the Saudi dietary guidelines was not significantly different between the CVD and non-CVD patients; however, the specific adherence scores of fruit ($p = 0.02$), olive oil ($p = 0.01$), and non-alcoholic beer ($p = 0.02$) were significantly higher in the non-CVD patients. The differences in CVD family history ($p = 0.02$) and adherence scores to specific groups/foods between the CVD and non-CVD patients may contribute to CVD risk in Saudi males. However, as the sample size of this study was small, further research is required to validate these findings.

Keywords: dietary intake; nutrition; cardiovascular disease

---

1. Introduction

Cardiovascular disease (CVD) is considered a major public health problem in Saudi Arabia [1,2], with an estimated 46% of all deaths attributed to CVD, and a 36% higher death rate in men compared to women [1]. The risk factors of CVD are characterized as modifiable factors such as diet, physical activity, obesity, and smoking, or non-modifiable factors such as aging, family history, and ethnicity [3–5]. The most important modifiable risk factor for CVD is diet [6–9]. Studies showed that a diet high in fruits, vegetables, whole grains as the major source of carbohydrates, and non-hydrogenated unsaturated fats as the main form of dietary fat, with adequate omega-3 fatty acids (monounsaturated fatty acid and polyunsaturated fatty acid), may reduce the risk of CVD [9–13]. Vitamins, minerals, fiber, and phenolic compounds are the main protective components found in fruit, vegetables, and whole grains with a functional role in reducing oxidative stress, inflammation, blood pressure, and improving insulin sensitivity and the lipoprotein profile [14–16]. In contrast, a diet containing a high intake of saturated fats, and refined and processed carbohydrates is linked with an increased CVD risk as a result of raised levels of blood glucose, total cholesterol, and low-density lipoprotein (LDL) cholesterol [17–22].

However, it is important to note that most of these nutritional studies evaluated the intake of a single nutrient, or small number of nutrients or food items in relation to risk of CVD. As individuals do not eat a single food or isolated nutrient, many researchers argued the importance of considering a holistic approach, investigating dietary patterns (combination of nutrients) rather than nutrient-based studies, when assessing health consequences [23–25]. Moreover, diet has a synergistic effect as it is a complex mixture of nutrients (within-food or across-food combinations), which could induce antagonistic effects on optimal health [23–25].

Dietary guidelines are a useful tool in public health policy, which can help reduce risk and prevent non-communicable diseases. Studies on dietary guideline adherence demonstrated their effectiveness in reducing the risk of disease, including CVD in multiple countries [24,26,27].

Current CVD research is dominated by studies that were conducted on Western populations with a paucity of research investigating the link between CVD and diet in Saudi Arabia [28,29]. Furthermore, to our knowledge no study used a holistic approach to consider the association of adherence to Saudi dietary guidelines with risk of CVD. We hypothesized that the non-adherence to the Saudi dietary guidelines could increase the risk of CVD in Saudi males.

2. Material and Methods

2.1. Study Design and Participants

A cross-sectional design study was performed at King Abdulaziz University Hospital (KAUH) in Jeddah, Saudi Arabia. Patients were recruited from the medical ward, surgical ward, and coronary care unit at KAUH. The inclusion criteria for CVD patients consisted of male cardiac patients, aged between 30–80 years old, as the prevalence of CVD among Saudi population increases after 30 years old [30]. The inclusion criteria for the non-CVD patients included male patients, in the same age range, who were free of CVD and had been admitted to the hospital for minor clinical conditions, including abdominal pain, eye surgery, and fever. Patients with liver, kidney, or respiratory disease, or any type of cancer diagnosis were excluded from recruitment to either group. Ethical approvals were obtained from the Faculty of Medicine Research Committee at King Abdulaziz University (Reference no. 307-14). All patients gave informed written consent.

2.2. The Saudi Dietary Guidelines

The message of the Saudi dietary guidelines is to follow a healthy diet including variety, balance, and moderation [31]. The main goals of these guidelines are (1) to improve health by promoting healthy eating options and encouraging physical activities; (2) to promote valuable food that high in nutrients such as foods rich in protein, fiber, vitamins, and minerals, and reduce foods of poor nutritional value such as foods high in salt, sugars, saturated fats, and hydrogenated fat; (3) to support the normal growth and development of infants, children, and adolescents; (4) to decrease the diseases related to diet in the Saudi community; and (5) to support physical activity.

To communicate the recommended food groups and serving sizes, the Saudi dietary guidelines are graphically represented in the form of a palm tree with the food groups distributed in the trunk and leaves of the palm in proportion to their recommended level of intake. The largest food group of bread and cereals was placed in the bottom big leaf of the palm and represents the most important source of carbohydrates (6–11 servings/day). Vegetables (3–5 servings/day) and fruits (2–4 servings/day) come next as they are high in vitamins and minerals. Milk and its products (2–4 servings/day) are the third largest group, which are essential sources of protein and calcium. The smallest group constitutes meat and beans (2–4 servings/day), and they are considered as sources of protein. Fat and sugar were in the smallest upper leaves of the palm (representing lower quantities); this shows the need to minimize their intake. Water was also added to the healthy food palm, due to the hot weather of

Saudi Arabia. As regular physical activity is essential, together with a balanced diet, the healthy food palm also recommends individuals to exercise for 30–60 min daily according to the individual's health status [31].

2.3. The Saudi Dietary Guideline Score

The score of adherence was given according to the Saudi dietary guidelines [31]. The ratings of the consumption of each food group (from 0 to 5 or the reverse) was adapted from Panagiotakos et al. (2006) [24]. The dietary adherence score included non-refined cereals and bread (whole bread, rice, pasta, and other grains), fruit, vegetables, legumes, fish, olive oil, non-alcoholic beer, meat and meat products, poultry, full-fat dairy products, sweets, and oils.

For the intake of food items assumed to be close to the Saudi dietary guidelines or higher (non-refined cereals, fruits, vegetables), we allocated a score of 0 when the individual stated no consumption, a score of 1 when they stated consumption of 1–4 servings/month, a score of 2 for 5–8 servings/month, a score of 3 for 9–12 servings/month, a score of 4 for 13–18 servings/month, and a score of 5 for more than 18 servings/month. Moreover, we included legumes, fish, and olive oil in this group after separating them from the meat and oil groups. Originally excluded from the Saudi guidelines, non-alcoholic beer was also added due to its health benefits for heart disease [32]. In contrast, for the intake of food items assumed to be limited in Saudi dietary guidelines (i.e., rare or monthly intake; meat and meat products, poultry, and full-fat dairy products), we allocated the scores on a reverse scale (i.e., 5, when individuals stated no intake, to 0, when they stated almost daily intake). Hence, the scores ranged from 0 to 60. Higher values of score show better adherence to the Saudi dietary guidelines (Table 1).

Table 1. The Saudi dietary guideline score.

No.	Food Groups	Frequency of Consumption (Servings/Month)					
		Never	1–4	5–8	9–12	13–18	>18
1	Non-refined cereals and bread [a]	0	1	2	3	4	5
2	Fruit [b]	0	1	2	3	4	5
3	Vegetable	0	1	2	3	4	5
4	Legumes	0	1	2	3	4	5
5	Fish	0	1	2	3	4	5
6	Olive oil	0	1	2	3	4	5
7	Non-alcoholic beer	0	1	2	3	4	5
8	Meat and meat products	5	4	3	2	1	0
9	Poultry	5	4	3	2	1	0
10	Full-fat dairy products	5	4	3	2	1	0
11	Sweets	5	4	3	2	1	0
12	Oils	5	4	3	2	1	0

[a] Whole-grain bread, rice, pasta etc. [b] Fresh (e.g., apple, oranges, banana, grapes, etc.) and dried fruit, including dates.

2.4. Procedure and Data Collection

An interview-administered survey consisting of four sections (demographics, anthropometrics, medical history, and a dietary assessment by food frequency questionnaire (FFQ)) was completed for each patient.

2.5. Demographics and Medical History

Personal information, including date of birth, gender, marital status, any medical diagnoses, and family history of cardiovascular diseases (whether at least one first-degree relative had CVD) was collected from the hospital electronic system at KAUH. Data regarding the education level, employment status, and tobacco use was collected during the interview process.

2.6. Anthropometric Measurements

The anthropometric measurements, including height, weight, waist circumference (WC), and body mass index (BMI) were performed according to standard procedures and carried out in the patient's ward. Patients were weighed in light clothing, without shoes, using a calibrated scale to the nearest 0.1 kg measured in kilograms. Height was measured to the nearest 0.1 cm. The BMI was computed as the fraction of weight to the squared height, with consideration for the cut-off for older adults (65 years old and older). The WC was taken at the level of the narrowest point between the lowest costal border and the iliac crest by the research team.

2.7. Estimation of Habitual Dietary Intake

The dietary intake was assessed using a 60-item food frequency questionnaire (FFQ). For each food item, patients were asked how frequently it was consumed during the last year on a daily, weekly, or monthly basis, along with the portion sizes. Food intake was grouped into food groups (milk and dairy products, fruits, vegetables, meats, rice, breads, beverages, legumes, and sweets). The average servings of each item consumed per week were calculated using Microsoft Excel version 1808 (Redmond, WA, USA).

2.8. Assessment of Blood Variables

Blood data were collected from the patients' records for the lipid profile (high-density lipoprotein (HDL), low-density lipoprotein (HDL), total cholesterol (TC), and triglycerides (TG)); blood glucose (fasting blood glucose (FBG) and glycated hemoglobin (HbA1c)); hemoglobin (HGB) and hematocrit (HCT); cardiac enzymes (aspartate aminotransferase (AST), creatine kinase (CK), lactate dehydrogenase (LDH), and cardiac troponin I (CTN-I)); and electrolytes (sodium (Na), potassium (K), and chloride (Cl)), according to the hospital policy.

2.9. Sample Size Calculation

This is a preliminary study to identify factors of interest and to develop a study protocol for a larger-scale study. No power calculation was conducted in this study due to the absence in Saudi literature of endpoints similar to the hypothesis proposed in this study. The data of this study serve as preliminary data to determine the needed sample size to achieve the aim of the study. We aimed to include 80 patients (40 with CVD and 40 without CVD disease).

2.10. Statistical Analysis

The statistical analysis was carried out using SPSS (version 23, SPSS, Inc, Chicago, IL, USA, 2015). A normality test was run on all data to determine if each dataset was well modeled by a normal distribution. Descriptive statistics are presented as medians and inter-quartile ranges (IQRs).

Linear regression models were performed using the diet score as an independent variable, with age, smoking history, educational level, diabetic history, and family history of CVD as covariates. Systolic blood pressure, serum total cholesterol, LDL, HDL, triglycerides, waist circumference, and body mass index were utilized as outcome variables. The results were presented as *b*-coefficients and standard error of the coefficient. Bonferroni correction was used due to multiple comparisons.

In addition, comparisons between the non-CVD patients and CVD patients were performed using a Mann–Whitney test for non-normally distributed data, and by paired *t*-test or two-sample *t*-test for normally distributed data. A chi-square test was used to compare the employment status and education level between the groups.

3. Results

3.1. Subject Characteristics

Eighty male patients were recruited for the study, aged between 30 and 80 years old. The demographic data for all individuals are presented in Table 2. There were no significant differences between non-CVD and CVD patients in terms of their age, education, or employment. However, there was a difference between non-CVD and CVD patients in terms of their family history, with significantly more CVD patients having at least one first-degree relative with CVD ($p = 0.02$; Table 3). The anthropometric characteristics, including blood pressure, weight, and BMI, were not significantly different between non-CVD and CVD patients (Table 4). The median BMI for both non-CVD and CVD patients was within the overweight cut-off range, with a value of 27.2 kg/m^2 (IQR 23.4–31.1) for the non-CVD patients and 25.7 kg/m^2 (IQR 23.4–27.7) for the CVD patients. The median waist circumference was within the normal range (< 102 cm) for both non-CVD (95.0 cm; IQR 85.8–100.0) and CVD patients (94.0 cm; IQR 90.0–98.3).

Table 2. Demographic data of the study participants.

Demographic Variable		All Patients (n = 80)		Non-CVD Patients (n = 40)		CVD Patients (n = 40)		p-Value *
		n	%	n	%	n	%	
Age (years)	30–55	36.0	45.0	21.0	52.5	15.0	37.5	0.09
	56–80	44.0	55.0	19.0	47.5	25.0	62.5	
Marital Status	Married	73.0	91.3	34.0	85.0	39.0	97.5	0.05
	Single	7.0	8.8	6.0	15.0	1.0	2.5	
Education	None	6.0	7.5	1.0	2.5	5.0	12.5	0.13
	Elementary	12.0	15.0	7.0	17.5	5.0	12.5	
	Intermediate	8.0	10.0	2.0	5.0	6.0	15.0	
	High School	32.0	40.0	20.0	50.0	12.0	30.0	
	University	22.0	27.5	10.0	25.0	12.0	30.0	
Employment	Employed	34.0	42.5	13.0	32.5	21.0	52.5	0.07
	Non-Employed	46.0	57.5	27.0	67.5	19.0	47.5	

n: number of patients, CVD: cardiovascular disease. * *p*-value between non-CVD and CVD patients.

Table 3. Family and smoking history of the study participants.

Variables		All Patients (n = 80)		Non-CVD Patients (n = 40)		CVD Patients (n = 40)		p-Value *
		n	%	n	%	n	%	
Family History	Negative	54.0	67.5	32.0	80.0	22.0	55.0	0.02
	Positive	26.0	32.5	8.0	20.0	18.0	45.0	
Diabetic	Yes	36.0	45.0	9	22.5	27	67.5	0.06
	No	44.0	55.0	31	77.5	13	32.5	
Smoking	Never	29.0	36.3	18.0	45.0	11.0	27.5	0.2
	Former >3 years	28.0	35.0	11.0	27.5	17.0	42.5	
	Former <3 years	7.0	8.8	2.0	5.0	5.0	12.5	
	Current	16.0	20.0	9.0	22.5	7.0	17.5	

n: number of patients; CVD: cardiovascular disease. * *p*-value between non-CVD and CVD patients.

Table 4. Anthropometric measurements of the study participants.

Variables	All Patients		Non-CVD Patients		CVD Patients		p-Value *
	Median	IQR	Median	IQR	Median	IQR	
Height (cm)	168.0 (n = 80)	160.0–172.2	165.0 (n = 40)	160.0–170.8	170.0 (n = 40)	160.0–170.8	0.6
Weight (kg)	70.0 (n = 80)	68.0–84.0	75.0 (n = 40)	67.5–86.0	70.0 (n = 40)	68.8–80.0	0.4
BMI (kg/m^2)	26.6 (n = 80)	23.4–29.4	27.2 (n = 40)	23.4–31.1	25.7 (n = 40)	23.4–27.7	0.3
WC (cm)	94.5 (n = 80)	88.2–99.7	95.0 (n = 40)	85.8–100.0	94.0 (n = 40)	90.0–98.3	0.5
Systolic BP	128.0 (n = 45)	117.5–140.0	128.0 (n = 26)	120.0–139.3	131.0 (n = 19)	119.5–142.0	0.1
Diastolic BP	76.0 (n = 45)	70.0–85.5	81.7 (n = 26)	75.0–87.8	70.0 (n = 19)	64.0–78.5	0.03
	n	%	n	%	n	%	
Underweight	7.0	8.8	2.0	5.0	5.0	12.5	
Normal weight	36.0	45.0	17.0	42.5	19.0	47.5	
Overweight	26.0	32.5	13.0	32.5	13.0	32.5	
Obese	11.0	13.8	8.0	20.0	3.0	7.5	

n: number of patients; CVD: cardiovascular disease; BMI: body mass index; BP: blood pressure; WC: waist circumference. * *p*-value between non-CVD and CVD patients.

3.2. Habitual Dietary Intake

The score of total adherence to the Saudi dietary guidelines was not significantly different between the non-CVD and CVD patients (Table 5); however, there were differences in adherence to dietary intake of some individual food groups. The specific adherence scores of fruit ($p = 0.02$), olive oil ($p = 0.01$), and non-alcoholic beer ($p = 0.02$) groups were significantly higher in the non-CVD patients (Table 5).

Table 5. The score of the adherence to the Saudi dietary guidelines.

	All Patients ($n = 80$)		Non-CVD Patients ($n = 40$)		CVD Patients ($n = 40$)		*p*-Value *
	Mean	SD	Mean	SD	Mean	SD	
Non-refined cereals and bread	1.2	2.1	1.5	2.3	1.0	1.9	0.29
Fruit	4.9	0.4	5.0	0.0	4.8	0.5	0.02
Vegetable	4.9	0.5	5.0	0.0	4.9	0.7	0.15
Legumes	3.6	1.6	3.6	1.6	3.6	1.7	0.98
Fish	2.8	1.6	2.7	1.6	3.0	1.5	0.37
Olive oil	2.7	2.1	3.2	2.1	2.1	2.0	0.01
Non-alcoholic beer	0.8	1.5	1.3	1.8	0.4	0.9	0.01
Meat and meat products	1.5	1.4	1.5	1.4	1.5	1.5	0.93
Poultry	1.5	1.6	1.2	1.5	1.8	1.6	0.06
Full-fat dairy products	0.1	0.6	0.1	0.3	0.2	0.7	0.17
Sweets	2.5	2.1	2.4	2.2	2.7	2.1	0.76
Oils	0.7	1.7	0.7	1.8	0.7	1.7	0.80
Total adherence to Saudi dietary guidelines	27.3	6.0	28.1	6.6	26.5	5.4	0.23

CVD: cardiovascular disease. * *p*-value between non-CVD and CVD patients.

Moreover, we evaluated the effect of the Saudi diet on various health outcomes such as systolic blood pressure, serum cholesterol, low-density lipoprotein, high-density lipoprotein, triglycerides, waist circumference, and body mass index. Table 6 shows the results of multiple linear regression after adjusting for age, smoking history, educational level, diabetic history, and family history of CVD. There were only significant associations found between the total adherence to Saudi dietary guideline score and serum total cholesterol and LDL.

Table 6. The association between different clinical and anthropometric factors (dependent) and total adherence to Saudi dietary guideline score (independent). Results of multiple linear regression analysis.

	β-Coefficient $\pm$ SE	*p*-Value
Model 1: Systolic blood pressure	-0.284 ± 0.508	0.579
Model 2: Serum cholesterol	-0.071 ± 0.023	0.004
Model 3: Low-density lipoprotein	-0.072 ± 0.028	0.012
Model 4: High-density lipoprotein	-0.021 ± 0.011	0.074
Model 5: Triglycerides	-0.032 ± 0.018	0.077
Model 6: Waist circumference	-0.308 ± 0.229	0.183
Model 7: Body mass index	-0.087 ± 0.102	0.399

All models were adjusted for age, smoking history, educational level, diabetic history, and family history of CVD. SE: Standard error.

3.3. Blood Variables

There were no significant differences in the lipid profile measurements of total cholesterol, triglycerides, or LDL between the non-CVD and CVD patients (Table 7). However, the HDL was significantly higher in the CVD patients compared to the non-CVD patients ($p = 0.03$). The HDL was 1.1 mmol/L (IQR 1.0–1.5) in the CVD patients and 1.0 mmol/L (IQR 0.6–1.1) in the non-CVD patients. There was no difference in hematological profile, with the exception of the median fasting blood glucose level, which was raised in all patients (normal range <5.6 mmol/L), but significantly higher ($p = 0.006$) in the CVD patients (7.5 mmol/L; IQR 6.2–11.7) than the non-CVD patients (6.1 mmol/L; IQR 5.1–7.2). In terms of the electrolyte and cardiac enzyme levels (Table 7), all biomarkers were non-significant between the non-CVD and CVD patients, with the exception of the potassium level ($p = 0.03$), which was within normal range (3.6–5.2 mmol/L) for all patients, but significantly higher in the CVD patients 4.1 mmol/L (IQR 3.5–4.4) than the non-CVD patients 3.7 mmol/L (IQR 3.5–4.0). In contrast, the chloride level was also within the normal range for all patients (98–106 mmol/L) but significantly lower ($p = 0.05$) in the CVD patients (99.0 mmol/L; IQR 94.8–102.0) compared to the non-CVD patients (101.0 mmol/L; IQR 98.0–104.0).

Table 7. Cardiovascular-related biomarkers.

Biomarkers	All patients		Non-CVD Patients		CVD Patients		p-Value *
	Median	IQR	Median	IQR	Median	IQR	
Lipids							
TC (mmol/L)	4.0 ($n = 80$)	3.0–4.6	4.0 ($n = 40$)	3.4–4.6	3.7 ($n = 40$)	3.0–4.6	0.7
TG (mmol/L)	1.3 ($n = 80$)	0.8–1.7	1.3 ($n = 40$)	0.8–1.9	1.2 ($n = 40$)	0.9–1.6	0.5
LDL (mmol/L)	2.7 ($n = 46$)	1.9–3.4	3.0 ($n = 18$)	2.3-3.6	2.6 ($n = 28$)	1.9-3.2	0.2
HDL (mmol/L)	1.1 ($n = 42$)	0.8–1.3	1.0 ($n = 17$)	0.6–1.1	1.1 ($n = 25$)	1.0–1.5	0.03
Hematological							
FBG (mmol/L)	6.5 ($n = 80$)	5.5–9.6	6.1 ($n = 40$)	5.1–7.2	7.5 ($n = 40$)	6.2–11.7	0.006
HbA1c (mmol/L)	7.4 ($n = 80$)	5.8–8.9	6.3 ($n = 40$)	5.4–7.4	8.2 ($n = 40$)	6.1–9.0	0.1
HGB (g/dl)	12.0 ($n = 80$)	10.0–13.6	12.3 ($n = 40$)	9.0–14.0	12.0 ($n = 40$)	10.3–13.1	0.7
HCT (%)	35.4 ($n = 80$)	30.1–40.5	36.5 ($n = 40$)	27.5–41.0	35.2 ($n = 40$)	31.8–39.3	0.8
Electrolytes							
Na (mmol/L)	137.0 ($n = 80$)	134.0–139.0	138.0 ($n = 40$)	135.0–140.0	137.0 ($n = 40$)	131.0–139.0	0.9
K (mmol/L)	3.9 ($n = 80$)	3.5–4.2	3.7 ($n = 40$)	3.5–4.0	4.1 ($n = 40$)	3.5–4.4	0.03
Cl (mmol/L)	99.5 ($n = 80$)	97.0–103.0	101.0 ($n = 40$)	98.0–104.0	99.0 ($n = 40$)	94.8–102.0	0.05
Cardiac Enzymes							
AST (U/L)	27.0 ($n = 69$)	19.0–41.3	26.0 ($n = 29$)	19.0–45.0	28.5 ($n = 40$)	19.0–40.5	0.12
CK (IU/L)	109.0 ($n = 52$)	52.0–214.0	95.5 ($n = 12$)	49.5–171.8	116.0 ($n = 40$)	63.0–249.0	0.4
LDH (U/L)	244.5 ($n = 51$)	191.8–304.0	215.0 ($n = 11$)	176.5–250.0	255.0 ($n = 40$)	212.0–310.0	0.1
CTN–I (ug/L)	0.1 ($n = 49$)	0.0–0.6	0.1 ($n = 09$)	0.0–0.3	0.1 ($n = 40$)	0.0–0.6	0.4

TC = total cholesterol; TG = triglycerides; LDL = low-density lipoprotein; HDL = high-density lipoprotein; FBG = fasting blood glucose; HbA1 = glycated hemoglobin; HGB = hemoglobin; HCT = hematocrit; Na = sodium; K = potassium; Cl = chloride; AST = aspartate aminotransferase; CK = creatine kinase; LDH = lactate dehydrogenase; CTN-I = cardiac troponin I. * p-value between non-CVD and CVD patients.

4. Discussion

This study was performed to test the hypothesis that the dietary patterns of Saudis may play a role in increasing the risk of CVD. To our knowledge, this is the first study that assesses the dietary intake using the adherence score to the Saudi dietary guidelines and its relationship to CVD in Saudi males living in Jeddah. As such, the data obtained from this study may be considered an important preliminary step in gaining an increased understanding of variables in the Saudi population that may affect their risk of CVD.

This study found a number of significant differences between the non-CVD and CVD patients that align with previously published studies. Firstly, the present study found that a family history of CVD was significantly higher in the CVD patients. This indicates the strong effect of genetics as a factor that could increase the risk of CVD. Studies showed that a family history is associated with an increase in CVD mortality across long-term follow-up [33].

Secondly, the evaluation of dietary habits using the adherence score to the Saudi dietary guidelines revealed that fruit, olive oil, and non-alcoholic beer were more highly consumed in the non-CVD patients than in the CVD patients. These food items are rich in polyphenols and dietary fiber, nutrients for which high levels of intake were previously associated with a decreased risk of developing CVD [34]. Moreover, we found that the consumption of non-refined cereals and breads was particularly low relative to recommendation. The high intake of refined carbohydrate is reported to increase the risk of type 2 diabetes and CVD [35]. The Saudi dietary guidelines are well publicized; however, more effort may be needed on education and promotion of the guidelines to reduce the risk of diseases including CVD.

Olive oil is the main source of fat in the Mediterranean diet and is linked with a lower mortality for CVD [18]. An olive-oil-rich diet is associated with enhanced lipoprotein metabolism and a reduction in oxidative damage, inflammation, blood pressure, endothelial dysfunction, and thrombosis [36]. A study by Guasch-Ferre et al, demonstrated that olive-oil intake, in particular the extra-virgin variety, decreased the risk of mortality and cardiovascular disease for individuals from Spain who were at high CVD risk [37]. Furthermore, a study by Carnevale et al. reported that olive oil advanced the post-prandial glucose and lipid profile in patients with impaired fasting glucose [38].

A study carried out by Woodside et al. found a strong correlation between the intake of fruits and vegetables and a reduction in the risk of developing coronary heart disease (CHD) [22]. Vegetables and fruits are a good source of nutrients, including vitamins, minerals, dietary fiber, and other biologically active compounds. These compounds have important mechanisms of action, including enhancing the immune system, reducing platelet aggregation, modulating cholesterol synthesis, reduction of blood pressure, and antioxidant, antibacterial, and antiviral effects [39].

The higher non-alcoholic beer consumption among the non-CVD patients may indicate that non-alcoholic beer could have a positive effect on heart health. It was reported that non-alcoholic beer can inhibit blood coagulation and platelet activation, which benefits the cardiovascular system without the negative effects of alcohol [32]. Despite the differences between non-CVD and CVD patients in their dietary habits, the lipid profile biomarkers, including total cholesterol, triglycerides, and LDL, were not significantly different. This is in contrast with the reported study by Rossouw, who showed that cholesterol levels are correlated with the risk of CHD, even at "normal" levels of cholesterol, in both men and women of all ages [40]. In addition, unpredictably, the levels of HDL were significantly higher in the CVD patients. The reason underlying this association is unknown, but one plausible explanation could be due to medications that were prescribed to CVD patients to control blood pressure, hyperlipidemia, and cardiac disease. These types of medications, such as niacin and atorvastatin, are known to enhance the lipid profile, and they were reported to increase HDL [41]. The current study also did not detect any significant differences between the non-CVD and CVD patients in the anthropometric measurements of weight, waist circumference, and BMI. This is in contrast with Alissa et al., who reported a strong significant relationship between BMI and the CVD risk in Saudi participants [29]. The inconsistency between these results could be due to differences in the sample size, which was smaller in this preliminary study. This study is the first to assess the adherence to the Saudi dietary guidelines among CVD male patients in Saudi Arabia. Currently, there is no validated food frequency questionnaire available specifically for the Saudi population; therefore, in this study, efforts were made to include food items that are more representative of the typical components of the Saudi diet. Furthermore, the analysis of adherence to the Saudi dietary guidelines was performed in parallel with the collection of blood biomarkers. As such, the data generated by this pilot study offer a unique insight into Saudi CVD populations, which may help in the planning and design of future studies to validate these findings. Further studies are now recommended to assess the association between the adherence to the Saudi dietary guidelines and the risk of CVD on a larger population sample. Moreover, as not all biomarker data of all for our patients were found in the patients' electronic system, the sample size calculation for future studies needs to consider the missing biomarker data of patients in the hospital electronic records when determining the power of their studies to allow for examining a more complete dataset of biomarkers.

5. Conclusions

The data from this preliminary study report a number of significant differences between non-CVD and CVD patients in terms of intake of particular food groups and CVD family history. These factors could be important contributors to the CVD risk in the Saudi population. Further research is now needed, using a larger sample size, in order to validate these findings and increase insight into the risk factors of the Saudi lifestyle that are associated with CVD.

Author Contributions: All authors made substantial contributions to the conception and study design. R.S.A, R.K.M, N.Y.E, and K.W.A carried out the data collation. A.A.A, R.S.A, R.K.M, and N.Y.E performed data analysis. R.S.A, R.K.M, and N.Y.E prepared the first draft of the manuscript. A.A.A, R.A.E.H.H, and K.W.A reviewed and edited the manuscript. All authors approved the final version of the manuscript.

Funding: This research received no external funding.

Acknowledgments: We would like to thank all our participants for their time and contribution in this study.

Conflicts of Interest: The authors declare no conflict of interest.

References

1. World Health Organization. Global Health Observatory: Cardiovascular Diseases-Country Statistics. Available online: https://www.who.int/cardiovascular_diseases/en/ (accessed on 04 August 2018).
2. Ahmed, A.M.; Hersi, A.; Mashhoud, W.; Arafah, M.R.; Abreu, P.C.; Al Rowaily, M.A.; Al-Mallah, M.H. Cardiovascular risk factors burden in Saudi Arabia: The Africa Middle East Cardiovascular Epidemiological (ACE) study. *J. Saudi Heart Assoc.* **2017**, *29*, 235–243. [CrossRef]
3. Petersen, S.E.; Sanghvi, M.M.; Aung, N.; Cooper, J.A.; Paiva, J.M.; Zemrak, F.; Fung, K.; Lukaschuk, E.; Lee, A.M.; Carapella, V.; et al. The impact of cardiovascular risk factors on cardiac structure and function: Insights from the UK Biobank imaging enhancement study. *PLoS ONE* **2017**, *12*, e0185114. [CrossRef]
4. Stamler, J.; Vaccaro, O.; Neaton, J.D.; Wentworth, D. Diabetes, other Risk-Factors, and 12-Yr Cardiovascular Mortality For Men Screened in The Multiple Risk Factor Intervention Trial. *Diabetes Care* **1993**, *16*, 434–444. [CrossRef] [PubMed]
5. Wong, N.D. Epidemiological studies of CHD and the evolution of preventive cardiology. *Nat. Rev. Cardiol.* **2014**, *11*, 276–289. [CrossRef]
6. Yusuf, S.; Hawken, S.; Ounpuu, S. Effect of potentially modifiable risk factors associated with myocardial infarction in 52 countries (the INTERHEART study): Case-control study. *Lancet* **2004**, *364*, 937–952. [CrossRef]
7. Hu, F.B.; Willett, W.C. Optimal diets for prevention of coronary heart disease. *JAMA* **2002**, *288*, 2569–2578. [CrossRef] [PubMed]
8. Hu, F. Optimal diet and lifestyle for prevention of coronary heart disease. *Atheroscler. Suppl.* **2003**, *4*, 6. [CrossRef]
9. Waskiewicz, A.; Szczesniewska, D.; Szostak-Wegierek, D.; Kwasniewska, M.; Pajak, A.; Stepaniak, U.; Kozakiewicz, K.; Tykarski, A.; Zdrojewski, T.; Zujko, M.E.; et al. Are dietary habits of the Polish population consistent with the recommendations for prevention of cardiovascular disease?—WOBASZ II project. *Kardiol. Pol.* **2016**, *74*, 969–977.
10. Panagiotakos, D.B.; Notara, V.; Kouvari, M.; Pitsavos, C. The Mediterranean and other Dietary Patterns in Secondary Cardiovascular Disease Prevention: A Review. *Curr. Vasc. Pharmacol.* **2016**, *14*, 442–451. [CrossRef] [PubMed]
11. Mahmood, D.; Jahan, K.; Habibullah, K. Primary prevention with statins in cardiovascular diseases: A Saudi Arabian perspective. *J. Saudi Heart Assoc.* **2015**, *27*, 179–191. [CrossRef] [PubMed]
12. Aljefree, N.; Ahmed, F. Association between dietary pattern and risk of cardiovascular disease among adults in the Middle East and North Africa region: A systematic review. *Food Nutr. Res.* **2015**, *59*, 27486. [CrossRef] [PubMed]
13. Vasilopoulou, A.; Galitsianos, I.; Fotiou, M.; Menexes, G.; Tsakoumaki, F.; Tsitlakidou, P.; Psirropoulos, D.; Michaelidou, A.M. An exploratory study of dietary intake patterns among adults diagnosed with cardiovascular risk factors. *Int. J. Food Sci. Nutr.* **2015**, *66*, 458–465. [CrossRef]
14. Conrad, Z.; Raatz, S.; Jahns, L. Greater vegetable variety and amount are associated with lower prevalence of coronary heart disease: National Health and Nutrition Examination Survey, 1999–2014. *Nutr. J.* **2018**, *17*, 67. [CrossRef]
15. Li, B.R.; Li, F.; Wang, L.F.; Zhang, D.F. Fruit and Vegetables Consumption and Risk of Hypertension: A Meta-Analysis. *J. Clin. Hypertens.* **2016**, *18*, 468–476. [CrossRef] [PubMed]

16. Aune, D.; Giovannucci, E.; Boffetta, P.; Fadnes, L.T.; Keum, N.; Norat, T.; Greenwood, D.C.; Riboli, E.; Vatten, L.J.; Tonstad, S. Fruit and vegetable intake and the risk of cardiovascular disease, total cancer and all-cause mortality-a systematic review and dose-response meta-analysis of prospective studies. *Int. J. Epidemiol.* **2017**, *46*, 1029–1056. [CrossRef] [PubMed]

17. Wang, X.; Ouyang, Y.; Liu, J.; Zhu, M.; Zhao, G.; Bao, W.; Hu, F.B. Fruit and vegetable consumption and mortality from all causes, cardiovascular disease, and cancer: Systematic review and dose-response meta-analysis of prospective cohort studies. *BMJ (Clin. Res. Ed.)* **2014**, *349*, g4490. [CrossRef] [PubMed]

18. Estruch, R.; Ros, E.; Salas-Salvado, J.; Covas, M.I.; Corella, D.; Aros, F.; Gomez-Gracia, E.; Ruiz-Gutierrez, V.; Fiol, M.; Lapetra, J.; et al. Primary Prevention of Cardiovascular Disease with a Mediterranean Diet Supplemented with Extra-Virgin Olive Oil or Nuts. *N. Engl. J. Med.* **2018**, *378*, e34. [CrossRef]

19. Menezes, R.; Rodriguez-Mateos, A.; Kaltsatou, A.; González-Sarrías, A.; Greyling, A.; Giannaki, C.; Andres-Lacueva, C.; Milenkovic, D.; Gibney, E.R.; Dumont, J.; et al. Impact of Flavonols on Cardiometabolic Biomarkers: A MetaAnalysis of Randomized Controlled Human Trials to Explore the Role of Inter-Individual Variability. *Nutrients* **2017**, *9*, 117. [CrossRef]

20. Trinity, J.D.; Pahnke, M.D.; Trombold, J.R.; Coyle, E.F. Impact of Polyphenol Antioxidants on Cycling Performance and Cardiovascular Function. *Nutrients* **2014**, *6*, 1273–1292. [CrossRef]

21. Zamora-Ros, R.; Knaze, V.; Lujan-Barroso, L.; Romieu, I.; Scalbert, A.; Slimani, N.; Hjartaker, A.; Engeset, D.; Skeie, G.; Overvad, K.; et al. Differences in dietary intakes, food sources and determinants of total flavonoids between Mediterranean and non-Mediterranean countries participating in the European Prospective Investigation into Cancer and Nutrition (EPIC) study. *Br. J. Nutr.* **2013**, *109*, 1498–1507. [CrossRef]

22. Woodside, J.; Young, I.S.; McKinley, M.C. Fruit and vegetable intake and risk of cardiovascular disease. *Proc. Nutr. Soc.* **2013**, *72*, 399–406. [CrossRef] [PubMed]

23. Tapsell, L.C.; Neale, E.P.; Satija, A.; Hu, F.B. Foods, Nutrients, and Dietary Patterns: Interconnections and Implications for Dietary Guidelines. *Adv. Nutr.* **2016**, *7*, 445–454. [CrossRef] [PubMed]

24. Panagiotakos, D.B.; Pitsavos, C.; Stefanadis, C. Dietary patterns: A Mediterranean diet score and its relation to clinical and biological markers of cardiovascular disease risk. *Nutr. Metab. Cardiovasc. Dis.* **2006**, *16*, 559–568. [CrossRef] [PubMed]

25. Martinez-Gonzalez, M.A.; Sanchez-Villegas, A. The emerging role of Mediterranean diets in cardiovascular epidemiology: Monounsaturated fats, olive oil, red wine or the whole pattern? *Eur. J. Epidemiol.* **2004**, *19*, 9–13. [CrossRef]

26. Reedy, J.; Krebs-Smith, S.M.; Miller, P.E.; Liese, A.D.; Kahle, L.L.; Park, Y.; Subar, A.F. Higher Diet Quality Is Associated with Decreased Risk of All-Cause, Cardiovascular Disease, and Cancer Mortality among Older Adults. *J. Nutr.* **2014**, *144*, 881–889. [CrossRef] [PubMed]

27. Russell, J.; Flood, V.; Rochtchina, E.; Gopinath, B.; Allman-Farinelli, M.; Bauman, A.; Mitchell, P. Adherence to dietary guidelines and 15-year risk of all-cause mortality. *Br. J. Nutr.* **2013**, *109*, 547–555. [CrossRef] [PubMed]

28. Alissa, E.M.; Bahjri, S.M.; Al-Ama, N.; Ahmed, W.H.; Starkey, B.; Ferns, G.A.A. Dietary vitamin A may be a cardiovascular risk factor in a Saudi population. *Asia Pac. J. Clin. Nutr.* **2005**, *14*, 137–144. [PubMed]

29. Eman, A.; Nabeel, A. Nutritional Intake and Cardiovascular Risk Factors in Saudi Subjects with Different Degrees of Atherosclerosis: A Case Control Study. *J. Nutr. Med. Diet. Care* **2015**, *1*, 008.

30. Rahman Al-Nuaim, A. High prevalence of metabolic risk factors for cardiovascular diseases among Saudi population, aged 30–64 years. *Int. J. Cardiol.* **1997**, *62*, 227–235. [CrossRef]

31. Ministry of Health. The Dietary Guidelines for Saudis. Available online: https://www.moh.gov.sa/en/HealthAwareness/Pages/SaudihealthFoodGuide.aspx (accessed on 16 March 2019).

32. Bassus, S.; Mahnel, R.; Scholz, T.; Wegert, W.; Westrup, D.; Kirchmaier, C.M. Effect of dealcoholized beer (Bitburger Drive) consumption on hemostasis in humans. *Alcohol. Clin. Exp. Res.* **2004**, *28*, 786–791. [CrossRef] [PubMed]

33. Bachmann, J.M.; Willis, B.L.; Ayers, C.R.; Khera, A.; Berry, J.D. Association Between Family History and Coronary Heart Disease Death Across Long-Term Follow-Up in Men The Cooper Center Longitudinal Study. *Circulation* **2012**, *125*, 3092–3098. [CrossRef] [PubMed]

34. Michalska, M.; Gluba, A.; Mikhailidis, D.P.; Nowak, P.; Bielecka-Dabrowa, A.; Rysz, J.; Banach, M. The role of polyphenols in cardiovascular disease. *Med. Sci. Monit.* **2010**, *16*, Ra110–Ra119. [PubMed]

35. Liu, S. Intake of refined carbohydrates and whole grain foods in relation to risk of type 2 diabetes mellitus and coronary heart disease. *J. Am. Coll. Nutr.* **2002**, *21*, 298–306. [CrossRef]

36. Covas, M.-I. Olive oil and the cardiovascular system. *Pharmacol. Res.* **2007**, *55*, 175–186. [CrossRef] [PubMed]

37. Guasch-Ferre, M.; Hu, F.B.; Martinez-Gonzalez, M.A.; Fito, M.; Bullo, M.; Estruch, R.; Ros, E.; Corella, D.; Recondo, J.; Gomez-Gracia, E.; et al. Olive oil intake and risk of cardiovascular disease and mortality in the PREDIMED Study. *BMC Med.* **2014**, *12*, 78. [CrossRef] [PubMed]

38. Carnevale, R.; Loffredo, L.; Del Ben, M.; Angelico, F.; Nocella, C.; Petruccioli, A.; Bartimoccia, S.; Monticolo, R.; Cava, E.; Violi, F. Extra virgin olive oil improves post-prandial glycemic and lipid profile in patients with impaired fasting glucose. *Clin. Nutr.* **2017**, *36*, 782–787. [CrossRef] [PubMed]

39. Lampe, J.W. Health effects of vegetables and fruit: Assessing mechanisms of action in human experimental studies. *Am. J. Clin. Nutr.* **1999**, *70* (Suppl. 3), 475s–490s. [CrossRef] [PubMed]

40. Rossouw, J.E. Serum cholesterol as a risk factor for coronary heart disease revisited. *S. Afr. J. Clin. Nutr.* **2015**, *28*, 34–37. [CrossRef]

41. Mani, P.; Rohatgi, A. Niacin Therapy, HDL Cholesterol, and Cardiovascular Disease: Is the HDL Hypothesis Defunct? *Curr. Atheroscler. Rep.* **2015**, *17*, 43. [CrossRef]

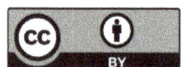

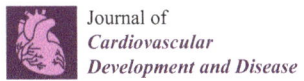

Journal of
*Cardiovascular
Development and Disease*

Brief Report

rs2569190A>G in *CD14* is Independently Associated with Hypercholesterolemia: A Brief Report

Ali Salami [1], Christy Costanian [2,3] and Said El Shamieh [4,*

[1] Rammal Hassan Rammal Research Laboratory, Physio-toxicity (PhyTox) Research Group,
    Lebanese University, Faculty of Sciences (V), Nabatieh 1700, Lebanon; a.salami@ul.edu.lb
[2] Faculty of Medicine, University of Ottawa, Ottawa 61350, ON K1G 5Z3, Canada; ccostani@uottawa.ca
[3] School of Medicine, Lebanese American University, Beirut 1102 2801, Lebanon
[4] Department of Medical Laboratory Technology, Faculty of Health Sciences, Beirut Arab University,
    Beirut 115020, Lebanon
*   Correspondence: s.elshamieh@bau.edu.lb; Tel.: +961-1-300110 (ext. 2721)

Academic Editor: Maurice Van den Hoff
Received: 5 September 2019; Accepted: 28 October 2019; Published: 30 October 2019

Abstract: Many studies have assessed the implication of *cluster of differentiation 14 (CD14)* molecules and its single nucleotide polymorphism rs2569190A>G with different complex diseases, such as diabetes and cardiovascular diseases (CVDs). In this study, we investigated the association of rs2569190A>G in *CD14* with cardiovascular disease risk factors (hypercholesterolemia and hypertension) in 460 individuals from the general Lebanese population (Middle Eastern multiethnic population). Using a multiple logistic regression model adjusted for six covariates (under additive and recessive assumptions), we found that the G allele of rs2569190 in *CD14* was associated with increased levels of total cholesterol (OR = 3.10, $p = 0.009$), low-density lipoprotein cholesterol (OR = 3.87, $p = 0.003$), and decreased levels of high-density lipoprotein cholesterol (OR = 0.38, $p = 0.001$). In contrast, no significant relationship was found with hypertension. Thus, we concluded that rs2569190G in *CD14* is associated with a higher risk of developing hypercholesterolemia.

Keywords: hypercholesterolemia; *cluster of differentiation 14*; rs2569190A>G; single nucleotide polymorphisms; association analysis

1. Introduction

According to the World Health Organization, cardiovascular diseases (CVDs) represent the most significant cause of death in humans globally [1]. Around 18 million people died because of CVDs in 2016, representing 31% of all deaths worldwide, most of which occur in low- and middle-income countries [1]. In addition to modifiable risk factors such as high cholesterol and triglyceride levels, diabetes, and high blood pressure (BP) levels [2], several studies have revealed an important impact of the innate immune system on the development or the progression of many CVDs [3]. The innate immune system present in multicellular living organisms gives an immediate defense capability against foreign bodies and pathogenic organisms such as viruses, bacteria, and fungi at first exposure [4]. This system depends on the recognition of pathogens by several families of extracellular receptors, such as the cluster of differentiation 14 (*CD14*), which is responsible for triggering innate immune responses and was first identified as marker of monocytes, before being defined as a coreceptor of toll-like receptors [5].

Many studies have assessed the role of *CD14*, especially at the molecular level, and established a link between the gene product and its single nucleotide polymorphisms (SNPs) with different complex diseases such as diabetes [6] and CVDs [7]. For example, the SNP rs2569190 in the promoter region of *CD14* has been found to be implicated in coronary artery disease through changing protein levels [8,9].

Furthermore, the A allele has been reported to be functional and enhances CD14 expression, and thus the host sensitivity, for exogenous or endogenous lipopolysaccharides [10]. More importantly, soluble *CD14* levels have shown strong, independent correlations with traditional cardio-metabolic risk factors and with subclinical measures of vascular disease (carotid wall thickness, ankle-brachial index, and body mass index) [7]. Based on all of the above, we hypothesize that rs2569190 in *CD14* could be associated with CVD risk factors such as hypercholesterolemia and hypertension (HTN). Therefore, the goal of our study was to investigate the association of rs2569190 in *CD14* with CVD risk factors in individuals from the general Lebanese population.

2. Materials and Methods

2.1. Study Population

The institutional review board of the Lebanese University approved the recruitment procedure and the genetic protocols (2182/28, on 16 December 2015). This cross-sectional study involved 460 unrelated Lebanese participants who were apparently healthy (free of chronic diseases; cardiovascular or cancer) individuals.

2.2. Clinical and Biological Data Collection

All measurements, including demographic, clinical, and biochemical measurements, were assessed as described previously [11]. Nuclear DNA was extracted from whole-blood samples according to the manufacturer's recommendations (QIAamp DNA blood mini kit, Qiagen, Hilden, Germany). Very briefly, 4 µg of total DNA from 200 µL of whole human blood was extracted through lysis and continuous spinning. A KASP genotyping assay (LGC group, Berlin, Germany) was used to genotype rs2569190A>G in *CD14*. Hypercholesterolemia was defined as an elevation of total cholesterol (Tchol) and/or low-density cholesterol (LDL-C) levels. Tchol and LDL-C were considered high if their values were ≥150 and ≥100 mg/dL, respectively. High-density cholesterol (HDL-C) levels were considered low if their values were ≤50 and ≤40 mg/dL in females and males, respectively. HTN was defined as systolic blood pressure ≥130 mmHg or diastolic ≥85 mmHg.

2.3. Statistical Analyses

SPSS statistical software version 24.0 [12] was used to perform all our statistical analyses except the power analysis. GPower 3.1.9.4 software [13] was used for the power analysis. Continuous variables were presented as mean value ± standard deviation, and categorical ones were shown as numbers and percentages. A chi-squared goodness-of-fit test was performed to determine if the genotypes of rs2569190A>G in *CD14* were in Hardy–Weinberg equilibrium (HWE).

To study the association between rs2569190A>G in *CD14* and hypercholesterolemia and HTN, a multivariate logistic regression model was used while correcting for different confounding factors (age, gender, body mass index, marital status, smoking, and physical activity). This analysis was performed under the assumption of additive (AA vs. GA vs. GG) and recessive models (AA and GA vs. GG). The sample size needed to reach a statistical power of at least 0.90 in a two-sided test with $\alpha = 0.05$ and an effect size of 0.2 was 409 individuals.

3. Results

3.1. Characteristics of the Studied Participants

The demographic characteristics of the study participants are shown in Table 1. The group of participants comprised 292 females (63.5%) and 168 males (36.5%). The mean age was 40.6 years old, and approximately 70% of the participants were married (Table 1). In addition, one-fourth of participants were smokers, and only a minority practiced physical exercise once per week (Table 1).

Table 1. Demographic characteristics of the study participants.

Characteristics	Participants (*n* = 460)
Age	40.60 ± 14.16
Gender *n* (%)	
Male	168 (36.5)
Female	292 (63.5)
Smoking status *n* (%)	
Nonsmoker	332 (72.2)
Past smoker	6 (1.3)
Current smoker	122 (26.5)
Marital Status *n* (%)	
Single	121 (26.3)
Married	321 (69.8)
Divorced	18 (3.9)
Physical Activity *n* (%)	
<1 per week	345 (75.0)
1 per week	52 (11.3)
≥2 per week	63 (13.7)

Values are arithmetic mean ± SD for continuous variables. Categorical variables are shown as numbers (*n*) and percentages (%). *n*: sample size.

Moreover, the clinical and genetic characteristics are shown in Table 2. Approximately 75% of the participants had high total cholesterol and LDL-C levels, and around half had low HDL-C.

Table 2. Clinical and genetic characteristics of the study participants.

Characteristics	Participants (*n* = 460)
BMI (Kg/m^2)	25.71 ± 4.98
Total cholesterol (mg/dL)	181.41 ± 40.94
High total cholesterol levels *n* (%)	351 (76.3)
LDL-C (mg/dL)	117.39 ± 33.52
High LDL-C levels *n* (%)	347 (75.4)
HDL-C (mg/dL)	45.53 ± 14.61
Low HDL-C levels *n* (%)	270 (58.7)
Triglycerides (mg/dL)	145.96 ± 124.34
High triglycerides levels *n* (%)	174 (37.8)
SBP (mmHg)	132.07 ± 15.89
DBP (mmHg)	67.82 ± 9.12
Hypertension *n* (%)	255 (55.4)
MAF of rs2569190G in *CD14*	0.41
AA *n* (%)	158 (34.3)
GA *n* (%)	224 (48.7)
GG *n* (%)	78 (17.0)

Values are arithmetic mean ± SD for continuous variables. Categorical variables are shown as number (*n*) and percentages (%). *n*: sample size. BMI: body mass index, LDL-C: low-density lipoprotein cholesterol, HDL-C: high-density lipoprotein cholesterol, SBP: systolic blood pressure, DBP: diastolic blood pressure, MAF: minor allele frequency, *CD14*: cluster of differentiation 14.

3.2. Association of rs2569190A>G in CD14 with Hypercholesterolemia

Our calculations showed that the minor allele in our population was the allele G, with a frequency of 0.41 (Table 2). In addition, the allelic frequencies were consistent with HWE ($p = 0.86$). Interestingly, the G allele of rs2569190 in *CD14* was associated with increased levels of Tchol (OR = 3.04, $p = 0.016$, Table 3) and LDL-C (OR = 3.83, $p = 0.006$, Table 3) and decreased levels of HDL-C (OR = 0.36, $p = 0.001$, Table 3). Similar results were also seen with a recessive genetic model. Age was positively associated with an increase in Tchol levels (OR = 2.06 and $p = 0.011$, Table 3) and LDL-C levels (OR = 2.22 and $p = 0.004$, Table 3). Similarly, smoking was significantly associated with an increase in Tchol levels (OR = 2.18, $p = 0.021$, Table 3) and LDL-C (OR = 1.88, $p = 0.050$, Table 3) and a decrease in HDL-C (OR = 0.41, $p = 0.001$, Table 3). Participants that practiced physical exercise once per week had decreased Tchol (OR = 0.27 and $p = 0.001$, Table 3), LDL-C (OR = 0.28 and $p = 0.001$, Table 3), and HDL-C (OR = 0.40 and $p = 0.017$, Table 3) levels.

Table 3. Multiple logistic regression analysis with hyperlipidemia and hypertension.

Variables	Total Cholesterol		LDL-Cholesterol		HDL-Cholesterol		Hypertension	
	OR (95% C.I.)	*p*	OR (95% C.I.)	*p*	OR (95% C.I.)	*p*	OR (95% C.I.)	*p*
rs2569190 AA	1		1		1		1	
GA	0.97 (0.57–1.63)	0.900	0.98 (0.59–1.64)	0.939	0.89 (0.56–1.43)	0.636	0.89 (0.56–1.40)	0.607
GG	3.04 (1.23–7.48)	0.016	3.83 (1.48–9.88)	0.006	0.36 (0.19–0.67)	0.001	0.67 (0.36–1.24)	0.203
rs2569190 AA and GA	1		1		1		1	
GG	3.10 (1.33–7.23)	0.009	3.87 (1.58–9.51)	0.003	0.38 (0.22–0.67)	0.001	0.72 (0.41–1.25)	0.186
Age								
<40	1		1		1		1	
≥40	2.06 (1.18–3.59)	0.011	2.22 (1.28–3.86)	0.004	1.58 (0.99–2.51)	0.056	0.73 (0.47–1.16)	0.181
Gender								
Male	1		1		1		1	
Female	1.21 (0.69–2.12)	0.503	0.98 (0.56–1.71)	0.931	1.17 (0.72–1.90)	0.523	0.46 (0.29–0.75)	0.002
BMI								
<25	1		1		1		1	
25–29.9	0.63 (0.34–1.15)	0.132	0.51 (0.28–0.93)	0.027	2.64 (1.50–4.65)	0.001	0.74 (0.44–1.26)	0.267
≥30	1.15 (0.56–2.34)	0.704	1.19 (0.58–2.43)	0.638	1.02 (0.57–1.80)	0.956	1.40 (0.78–2.51)	0.256
Marital status								
Single	1		1		1		1	
Married	0.60 (0.31–1.15)	0.124	0.83 (0.44–1.56)	0.566	0.75 (0.43–1.30)	0.306	0.70 (0.41–1.22)	0.206
Divorced	0.76 (0.21–2.76)	0.681	1.06 (0.29–3.83)	0.935	2.06 (0.57–7.47)	0.271	0.33 (0.10–1.07)	0.065
Smoking status								
Non smoker	1		1		1		1	
Past smoker	0.71 (0.11–4.62)	0.720	0.72 (0.11–4.72)	0.735	0.63 (0.11–3.67)	0.607	0.17 (0.03–1.13)	0.067
Current smoker	2.18 (1.12–4.21)	0.021	1.88 (0.99–3.53)	0.050	0.41 (0.24–0.68)	0.001	0.74 (0.45–1.22)	0.233
Physical activity								
<1 per week	1		1		1		1	
1 per week	0.27 (0.13–0.58)	0.001	0.28 (0.13–0.60)	0.001	0.40 (0.19–0.85)	0.017	0.99 (0.48–2.04)	0.971
≥2 per week	0.69 (0.33–1.41)	0.304	1.27 (0.59–2.74)	0.536	0.57 (0.30–1.11)	0.100	0.90 (0.48–1.70)	0.752

OR: odds ratio, C.I: confidence interval, BMI: body mass index.

4. Discussion

The results of the current study indicated that rs2569190A>G in *CD14* was associated with increased levels of Tchol and LDL-C and decreased levels of HDL-C. This might point to a possible role for *CD14* in the pathophysiology of hypercholesterolemia.

Human *CD14* is located on the long arm of chromosome 5 (q23-31), which encodes the membrane (m)*CD14*, binds to lipopolysaccharides, and activates various TLRs and downstream proinflammatory pathways [14]. Additionally, *CD14* exists in a soluble form (s)*CD14* [15]. In response to interleukin-6, its expression is increased; therefore, it is regarded as an acute phase protein [16]. Of interest, Reiner et al. reported that (s)*CD14* was positively correlated with LDL-C and HTN and negatively correlated with HDL-C [7]. When combined with our results, the above suggests that the *CD14* gene and protein might be implicated in CVDs.

J. Cardiovasc. Dev. Dis. **2019**, *6*, 37

Increasing experimental evidence is suggesting that rs2569190A>G in the *CD14* promoter could contribute to the genetic etiology of human atherosclerosis [17,18]. This SNP was shown to be functional and increase the transcriptional activity of *CD14* [10], which leads to higher (m)*CD14* protein levels and an increased risk of myocardial infarction [17,18].

The current study is not the first to find a link between elements of the innate immune system (*CD14*) and CVD risk factors, since activated innate immune system elements and dysfunction in metabolic pathways could lead to the chronic inflammation and pathologic conditions associated with CVDs [19]. Benachour et al. reported that the expression of the antimicrobial peptide *LL-37* (a component of the immune system) was positively correlated with CVD risk factors such as systolic BP and triglyceride levels, and negatively with plasma levels of HDL-C, in a sample of 90 apparently healthy men [20]. Another component of the innate immune system that has a noteworthy association with CVD risk factors is the human formyl peptide receptor 1 (*FPR1*) [21]. We have previously identified that, in 1012 French middle-aged adults equally divided between healthy and hypertensive individuals, *FPR1* C32T (rs5030878) is associated with increased BP levels [21].

It is noteworthy to mention that a Hardy–Weinberg equilibrium for rs2569190 was found despite the participants belonging to the Middle Eastern population, where consanguinity rates are higher than in European populations. This might be explained by the fact that the majority of the studied individuals came from a northern large city (not villages), making mating less consanguineous and more random.

5. Conclusions

In conclusion, our results indicate that rs2569190A>G in *CD14* is positively associated with increased Tchol and LDL-C and negatively correlated with HDL-C. This link with hypercholesterolemia might highlight that rs2569190A>G in *CD14* could be implicated in the pathophysiology of hypercholesterolemia. Further studies are needed in order to highlight its possible role in the pathogenesis of CVDs.

Author Contributions: Conceptualization, S.E.S. and C.C.; Data curation, A.S.; Formal analysis, A.S.; Methodology, S.E.S.; Project administration, S.E.S.; Software, A.S.; Validation, A.S., C.C., and S.E.S.; Visualization, A.S. and S.E.S.; Writing—original draft, A.S. and S.E.S.; Writing—review and editing, A.S. and S.E.S.

Funding: The present work was funded with support from the Lebanese University, Beirut, Lebanon.

Conflicts of Interest: The authors declare no conflicts of interest.

References

1. World Health Organization. *A Report about Cardiovascular Diseases*; Avenue Appia: Geneva, Switzerland, 17 May 2017.
2. Upadhyay, R.K. Emerging risk biomarkers in cardiovascular diseases and disorders. *J. Lipids* **2015**, *2015*, 971453. [CrossRef] [PubMed]
3. Frantz, S.; Falcao-Pires, I.; Balligand, J.L.; Bauersachs, J.; Brutsaert, D.; Ciccarelli, M.; Dawson, D.; de Windt, L.J.; Giacca, M.; Hamdani, N.; et al. The innate immune system in chronic cardiomyopathy: A European Society of Cardiology (ESC) scientific statement from the Working Group on Myocardial Function of the ESC. *Eur. J. Heart Fail.* **2018**, *20*, 445–459. [CrossRef] [PubMed]
4. Turvey, S.E.; Broide, D.H. Innate immunity. *J. Allergy Clin. Immunol.* **2010**, *125*, S24–S32. [CrossRef] [PubMed]
5. Baumann, C.L.; Aspalter, I.M.; Sharif, O.; Pichlmair, A.; Bluml, S.; Grebien, F.; Bruckner, M.; Pasierbek, P.; Aumayr, K.; Planyavsky, M.; et al. CD14 is a coreceptor of Toll-like receptors 7 and 9. *J. Exp. Med.* **2010**, *207*, 2689–2701. [CrossRef] [PubMed]
6. Fernandez-Real, J.M.; Perez del Pulgar, S.; Luche, E.; Moreno-Navarrete, J.M.; Waget, A.; Serino, M.; Sorianello, E.; Sanchez-Pla, A.; Pontaque, F.C.; Vendrell, J.; et al. CD14 modulates inflammation-driven insulin resistance. *Diabetes* **2011**, *60*, 2179–2186. [CrossRef]
7. Reiner, A.P.; Lange, E.M.; Jenny, N.S.; Chaves, P.H.; Ellis, J.; Li, J.; Walston, J.; Lange, L.A.; Cushman, M.; Tracy, R.P. Soluble CD14: Genomewide association analysis and relationship to cardiovascular risk and mortality in older adults. *Arterioscler. Thromb. Vasc. Biol.* **2013**, *33*, 158–164. [CrossRef]

8. Konstantinidou, M.K.; Goutas, N.; Vlachodimitropoulos, D.; Chaidaroglou, A.; Stefanou, D.; Poumpouridou, N.; Mastorakou, R.; Gazouli, M.; Kyparissopoulos, D.; Spiliopoulou, C. TLR-4 and CD14 Genotypes and soluble cd14: Could they predispose to coronary atherosclerosis? *J. Cardiovasc. Dev. Dis.* **2016**, *3*, 9. [CrossRef]

9. Raza, S.T.; Abbas, S.; Eba, A.; Karim, F.; Wani, I.A.; Rizvi, S.; Zaidi, A.; Mahdi, F. Association of COL4A1 (rs605143, rs565470) and CD14 (rs2569190) genes polymorphism with coronary artery disease. *Mol. Cell. Biochem.* **2018**, *445*, 117–122. [CrossRef]

10. Mertens, J.; Bregadze, R.; Mansur, A.; Askar, E.; Bickeboller, H.; Ramadori, G.; Mihm, S. Functional impact of endotoxin receptor CD14 polymorphisms on transcriptional activity. *J. Mol. Med. (Berl.)* **2009**, *87*, 815–824. [CrossRef] [PubMed]

11. Assaad, S.; Costanian, C.; Jaffal, L.; Tannous, F.; Stathopoulou, M.G.; El Shamieh, S. Association of TLR4 Polymorphisms, Expression, and Vitamin D with helicobacter pylori Infection. *J. Pers. Med.* **2019**, *9*, 2. [CrossRef] [PubMed]

12. IBM Corp. *IBM SPSS Statistics for Windows, Version 24.0*; IBM Corp: Armonk, NY, USA, 2016.

13. Faul, F.; Erdfelder, E.; Lang, A.G.; Buchner, A. G*Power 3: A flexible statistical power analysis program for the social, behavioral, and biomedical sciences. *Behav. Res. Methods* **2007**, *39*, 175–191. [CrossRef] [PubMed]

14. Wright, S.D.; Ramos, R.A.; Tobias, P.S.; Ulevitch, R.J.; Mathison, J.C. CD14, a receptor for complexes of lipopolysaccharide (LPS) and LPS binding protein. *Science* **1990**, *249*, 1431–1433. [CrossRef] [PubMed]

15. Bazil, V.; Baudys, M.; Hilgert, I.; Stefanova, I.; Low, M.G.; Zbrozek, J.; Horejsi, V. Structural relationship between the soluble and membrane-bound forms of human monocyte surface glycoprotein CD14. *Mol. Immunol.* **1989**, *26*, 657–662. [CrossRef]

16. Bas, S.; Gauthier, B.R.; Spenato, U.; Stingelin, S.; Gabay, C. CD14 is an acute-phase protein. *J. Immunol.* **2004**, *172*, 4470–4479. [CrossRef] [PubMed]

17. Unkelbach, K.; Gardemann, A.; Kostrzewa, M.; Philipp, M.; Tillmanns, H.; Haberbosch, W. A new promoter polymorphism in the gene of lipopolysaccharide receptor CD14 is associated with expired myocardial infarction in patients with low atherosclerotic risk profile. *Arter. Thromb Vasc. Biol.* **1999**, *19*, 932–938. [CrossRef] [PubMed]

18. Hubacek, J.A.; Rothe, G.; Pit'ha, J.; Skodova, Z.; Stanek, V.; Poledne, R.; Schmitz, G. C(-260)–>T polymorphism in the promoter of the CD14 monocyte receptor gene as a risk factor for myocardial infarction. *Circulation* **1999**, *99*, 3218–3220. [CrossRef] [PubMed]

19. Mann, D.L. The emerging role of innate immunity in the heart and vascular system: For whom the cell tolls. *Circ. Res.* **2011**, *108*, 1133–1145. [CrossRef] [PubMed]

20. Benachour, H.; Zaiou, M.; Samara, A.; Herbeth, B.; Pfister, M.; Lambert, D.; Siest, G.; Visvikis-Siest, S. Association of human cathelicidin (hCAP-18/LL-37) gene expression with cardiovascular disease risk factors. *Nutr. Metab. Cardiovasc. Dis.* **2009**, *19*, 720–728. [CrossRef] [PubMed]

21. El Shamieh, S.; Herbeth, B.; Azimi-Nezhad, M.; Benachour, H.; Masson, C.; Visvikis-Siest, S. Human formyl peptide receptor 1 C32T SNP interacts with age and is associated with blood pressure levels. *Clin. Chim. Acta* **2012**, *413*, 34–38. [CrossRef] [PubMed]

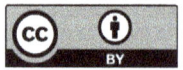

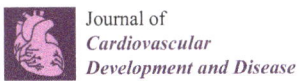

Journal of
Cardiovascular
Development and Disease

MDPI

Review

Association Between Smoking Hookahs (Shishas) and Higher Risk of Obesity: A Systematic Review of Population-Based Studies

Reem Baalbaki, Leila Itani, Lara El Kebbi, Rawan Dehni, Nermine Abbas, Razan Farsakouri, Dana Awad, Hana Tannir, Dima Kreidieh, Dana El Masri and Marwan El Ghoch *

Department of Nutrition and Dietetics, Faculty of Health Sciences, Beirut Arab University, P.O. Box 11-5020 Riad El Solh, Beirut 11072809, Lebanon; reembaalbaki1998@gmail.com (R.B.); l.itani@bau.edu.lb (L.I.); larakebbe@gmail.com (L.E.K.); rawan-dehni@hotmail.com (R.D.); nermine.abbas7@gmail.com (N.A.); razane.fa@hotmail.com (R.F.); dana_awad@outlook.com (D.A.); hana.tannir@bau.edu.lb (H.T.); d.kraydeyeh@bau.edu.lb (D.K.); dana.masri@bau.edu.lb (D.E.M.)
* Correspondence: m.ghoch@bau.edu.lb; Tel.: +9611300110 (ext. 2332)

Received: 28 May 2019; Accepted: 14 June 2019; Published: 16 June 2019

Abstract: The American Heart Association has published a scientific statement on the effect of hookah smoking on health outcomes; nevertheless, hookah smoking continues to be popular worldwide, especially among the young. Recent reports mention a potential link between hookah smoking and obesity; however, uncertainties still surround this issue. The aim of the current study was to conduct a systematic review to clarify whether hookah smoking is associated with a higher risk of obesity among the general population. This study was conducted in compliance with the preferred reporting items for systematic reviews and meta-analyses (PRISMA) guidelines, and data were collated by means of a meta-analysis and a narrative synthesis. Of the 818 articles retrieved, five large-population and low-bias studies comprising a total of 16,779 participants met the inclusion criteria and were reviewed. All included studies reported that, regardless of gender, hookah smoking increases the risk of obesity among all ages and observed an association between the two after a correction for several confounders or reported a higher prevalence of obesity among hookah smokers. This was confirmed by the meta-analysis. Therefore, hookah smoking seems to be associated with a higher risk of obesity. Public health policymakers should be aware of this for the better management of obesity and weight-related comorbidities.

Keywords: obesity; hookah; overweight; shisha; abdominal obesity; weight management; treatment

---

1. Introduction

The hookah, also known as a water pipe, narghile, arghile, or shisha, was invented in the 16th century as an attempt to purify smoke through water [1]. Nowadays hookah smoking is becoming popular in developing countries as well as in Western countries, especially among the young [2–4]. In fact, many hookah smokers consider this practice less harmful than smoking cigarettes because of the misconception that inhaling smoke containing fruit flavours, (i.e., apple, orange, grapes, etc.) through hookah water is less toxic [5]. Strong evidence supports the association between hookah smoking and several chronic diseases as well as a high risk of cancer [6–14] to the extent where it is considered a serious public health problem. This caused the American Heart Association to issue a scientific statement on hookah smoking and the increased risk of cardiovascular disease [15].

On the other hand, obesity is another increasing health problem. It is becoming one of the most serious conditions worldwide, known to be associated with several comorbidities that lead to an increase in disability, morbidity, and mortality [16–21]. Recently, reputable magazine reports have mentioned a potential association between obesity and hookah smoking; however, this is still uncertain [22]. Moreover, to the best of our knowledge, no systematic review considering this issue as a primary outcome has yet been conducted in order to provide a valid interpretation of the evidence published to date based on a systematic review and a meta-analysis. In light of these considerations, we hypothesised an association between hookah smoking and a higher risk of obesity and aimed to systematically review the published literature on this topic in accordance with the PICO process [23], as detailed below:

P—Population: adolescents and adults of both genders [24]; I—Intervention: active hookah smoking; C—Comparison: hookah-smoking group vs. nonsmoking group (when available) or hookah-smoking group vs. cigarette-smoking group (when available); and O—Outcome: obesity, however defined, based on international guidelines, (e.g., BMI, BMI percentiles, waist circumference, body fat percentage, etc.).

2. Methods

The current study was completed according to the Preferred Reporting Items for the Systematic reviews and Meta-Analyses (PRISMA) guidelines [25,26] and registered in the PROSPERO registry, York, UK—Association between smoking shisha, obesity, and related comorbidities: a systematic review (CRD42019129389) [27].

2.1. Inclusion and Exclusion Criteria

All studies evaluating hookah smoking and obesity were included, provided they met the following criteria: (i) they were written in English, (ii) they were original articles, and (iii) they related to prospective or retrospective observational (analytical or descriptive), experimental, or quasi-experimental controlled or noncontrolled studies. Reviews or non-original articles (e.g., case reports, editorials, letters to editors, or book chapters) were excluded.

2.2. Information Source and Search Strategy

The literature search was designed and performed independently in duplicate by two of the authors: the principal and the senior investigator. The PubMed/MEDLINE database was systematically screened using the following MeSH terms: #1 = Obesity, #2 = Hookah, #3 = Water pipe, #4 = Narghile, #5 = Arghile, and #6 = Shisha, together with the combinations #1 AND #2 OR #3 OR #4 OR #5 OR #6. In addition, a manual search was carried out to retrieve other articles that had not been identified via the initial search strategy. The publication date was not considered as an exclusion criterion for the purposes of this review.

2.3. Study Selection

Two authors independently screened the resulting articles for their methodologies and appropriateness for inclusion. All the included studies underwent a risk-of-bias assessment according to the 10-item quality assessment checklist for prevalence studies adapted by Hoy and colleagues, in which a total score of 0–3 indicates a low risk of bias, a score of 4–6 indicates a moderate risk of bias, and a score of 7–9 indicates a high risk of bias [28]. Consensus discussions were used to resolve disagreements between reviewers.

2.4. Data Collection Process and Data Items

The title and abstract of each paper were firstly assessed by two independent authors for language suitability and subject-matter relevance, and the studies selected were assessed in terms of their appropriateness for inclusion and the quality of the method. Those studies passing both rounds of screening are shown in Table 1.

Table 1. Summary of the included studies.

Study	Design	Country	Sample	Age	Primary Outcome	Findings
Shafique et al. 2012	Population-based study	Pakistan	Total = 2032 HS = 325 of both genders	30–75 years	• Association between HS and metabolic syndrome and components	• Metabolic syndrome was significantly higher among HS (33.1%) compared to NS. • HS were 3 times more likely to have metabolic syndrome compared with NS. • HS have significantly more hypertriglyceridemia, hyperglycaemia, hypertension, and abdominal obesity with respect to non-HS.
Ward et al. 2015	Population-based study	Syria	Total = 2536, NS = 2134, former HS = 116, 251 non-daily HS = 251, daily HS = 35 of both genders	≥18 years	• Associations of HS use status with BMI and obesity status	• Daily HS have nearly 2 BMI units greater than NS and had nearly three times the risk of having obesity.
Saffar Soflaei et al. 2018	Population-based study	Iran	Total = 9840, NS = 6742, Ex-smoker = 976 CS = 864, HS = 1067, MS = 41 of both genders	35–65 years	Association between HS and obesity, cardiovascular disease, diabetes mellitus, metabolic syndrome, and dyslipidemia	• A positive association between HS and metabolic syndrome, diabetes, obesity, and dyslipidemia was not established in CS.
Alomari et al. 2018	Population-based study	Jordan	Total = 2313 of both genders	In grades 7–10	• Associations of obesity with HS	• HS when compared to nonusers and who smoked hookah weekly had twofold greater odds of having obesity than nonsmokers.
Hasni et al. 2018	Population-based study	Tunisia	Total = 58, HS = 29, NS = 29 only males	25–45 years	• Comparison in the biochemical data and the metabolic profile between HS and nonsmokers	• The mean BMI in HS was significantly higher when compared with that of nonsmokers and had a higher prevalence of obesity and abdominal obesity.

HS = hookah smokers; NS = nonsmokers; CS = cigarette-smokers; BMI = body mass index.

2.5. Data Synthesis

The studies that met the inclusion criteria have been presented as a narrative synthesis [29,30]. Subsequently, a meta-analysis was conducted, detecting the association between hookah smoking and the risk of obesity, however expressed, using Review Manager 5 (RevMan 5.3. Copenhagen, Denmark) software developed by and for the Cochrane collaboration [31]. A random effects model was used to calculate the pooled relative risk and the 95% CI.

3. Results

The initial search retrieved 818 papers. After the first round of screening (titles and abstracts), 408 papers were excluded on the following grounds: They were not in English or did not study humans, or the abstracts and full texts were not available. The second round of screening excluded articles (n = 326) that represented an inappropriate type of paper, were not an original research article, (e.g., reviews, letters to editors, book chapters, and case reports), or were not related to smoking or obesity and related comorbidities. Of the remaining 84 articles dealing with smoking and health status, a further 79 papers were excluded on the following grounds: They were on smoking but not on hookahs, they considered health outcomes other than obesity and related comorbidities (e.g., cancer, respiratory diseases, acute effects of hookah-smoking such as heart rate, etc.), or other factors, (e.g., they were conducted in clinical settings rather than in the general population). Thus, at the end of the screening process, five articles were available for systematic review, narrative synthesis, and meta-analysis (Figure 1). According to the quality assessment checklist for prevalence studies (n = 5), these studies had a low risk of bias (mean score of 1.2 points) (Table 2).

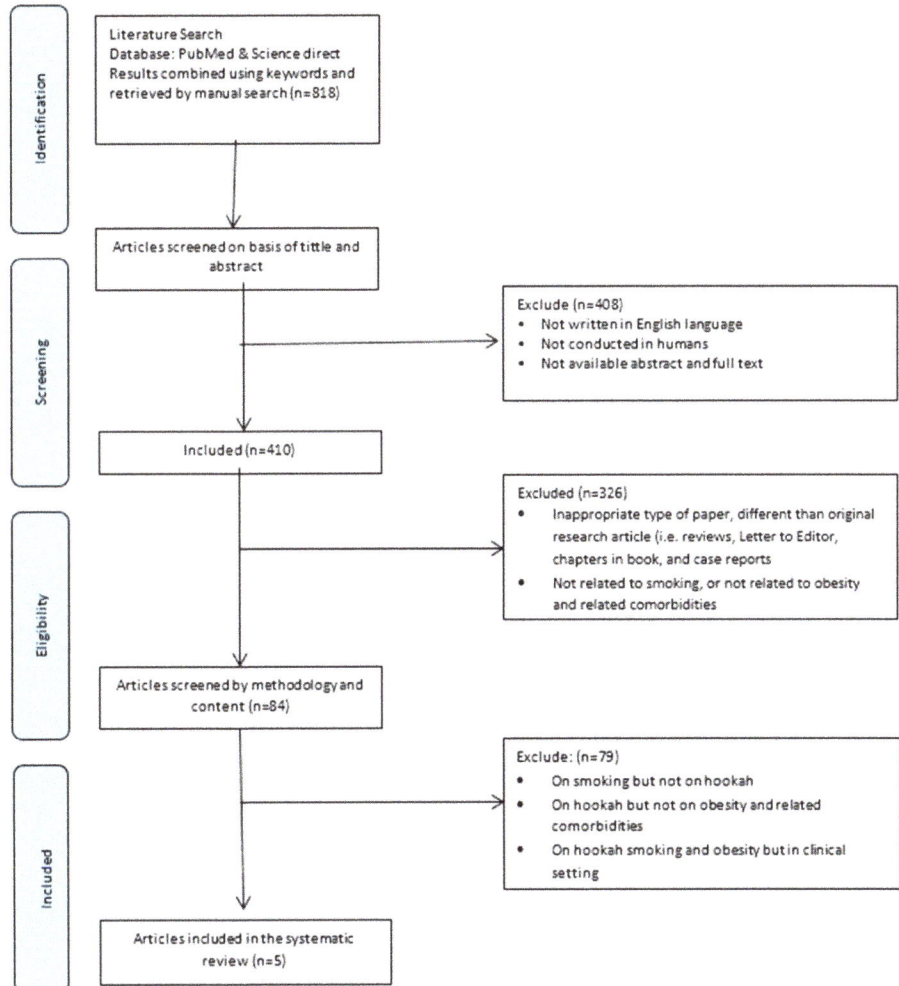

Figure 1. The flowchart summarizing the study selection procedure.

J. Cardiovasc. Dev. Dis. **2019**, *6*, 23

Table 2. Quality assessment checklist for prevalence studies.

	Shafque 2012	Ward 2015	Saffar Sofaei 2018	Alomari 2018	Hasni 2018
Was the study's target population a close representation of the national population in relation to relevant variables, e.g., age, sex, occupation?	0	0	0	0	1
Was the sampling frame a true or close representation of the target population?	0	0	0	0	1
Was some form of random selection used to select the sample, OR was a census undertaken?	0	0	0	1	1
Was the likelihood of nonresponse bias minimal?	0	1	0	0	1
Were data collected directly from the subjects as opposed to a proxy?	0	0	0	0	0
Was an acceptable case definition used in the study?	0	0	0	0	0
Was the study instrument that measured the parameter of interest shown to have reliability and validity (if necessary)?	0	0	0	0	0
Was the same mode of data collection used for all subjects?	0	0	0	0	0
Were the numerator(s) and denominator(s) for the parameter of interest appropriate?	0	0	0	0	0
Summary on the overall risk of study	0	1	0	1	4

Yes = 0; No = 1; Total score 0–3 = low risk of bias; 4–6 = moderate risk of bias; 7–9 = high risk of bias

3.1. Narrative Synthesis

In 2012, Shafique et al. [32] conducted a cross-sectional population-based study to investigate the association between hookah smoking and metabolic syndrome as a primary outcome. The sample included 2032 individuals, of which 325 were current hookah smokers. Metabolic syndrome was significantly higher among the current hookah smokers (33.1%) compared to nonsmokers (14.8%); the former were three times more likely to have metabolic syndrome compared with nonsmokers after an adjustment for confounders. Moreover, the definition of obesity was based on waist circumference. For abdominal obesity, the authors used a South Asian-specific cutoff of ≥ 90 cm waist circumference for males and of ≥ 80 cm for females [33]. In fact, hookah smokers had a significantly greater waist circumference (84.7 ± 12.6 vs. 80.6 ± 11.8; $p < 0.01$), and a logistic regression analysis showed that hookah smokers were significantly more likely to show abdominal obesity (OR 1.93, 95% CI 1.52–2.45).

In 2015, Ward et al. [34] conducted a population-based household study among 2536 adults (age ≥ 18 years) and examined the associations between hookah smoking and BMI and obesity status (BMI ≥ 30 kg/m^2). Of the total sample 2134 had never smoked a hookah, 116 were former smokers, 251 were current non-daily smokers, and 35 were current daily smokers. The mean BMI of the entire sample was 30.2 ± 6.3 kg/m^2. The authors found that daily hookah smokers had a BMI nearly 2 units greater than nonsmokers and had nearly three times the risk of obesity.

In 2018, Saffar Soflaei et al. [35] published a large population study with a total of 9840 subjects living in the city of Mashad (Iran), allocated to five different groups: nonsmokers (n = 6742), ex-smokers (n = 976), cigarette smokers (n = 864), hookah smokers (n = 1067), and cigarette and hookah smokers (n = 41). The authors found a significant association between hookah smoking (not cigarette-smoking) and obesity. They concluded that, in contrast to the common belief that the hookah eliminates the toxicity of tobacco compared with cigarettes, the adverse effects of hookah smoking could be even greater than those of cigarette smoking. In fact, in this study, the prevalence of obesity was significantly higher in hookah smokers compared with nonsmokers and even cigarette smokers.

In 2018, Alomari et al. [36] studied the associations between obesity and hookah smoking among 2313 adolescents of both genders at public schools in grades seven to 10 in Jordan using a cross-sectional design. The BMI percentile z-scores were calculated to determine weight-status categories, and obesity was defined as the 95th percentile or greater. Of the entire sample, 279 (12.1%) were obese. The authors found that body weight and age- and gender specific BMI were higher for hookah smokers compared to nonsmokers and that those who smoked a hookah weekly had double the odds of being obese compared to nonsmokers (OR = 2.14; 95% CI = 1.08–4.21; $p = 0.028$). They concluded that hookah use and dual use are associated with greater obesity, BMI, and body weight among Jordanian adolescents.

In 2018, Hasni et al. [37] undertook a small population study that aimed to compare the biochemical and metabolic profiles of hookah smokers and nonsmokers in 58 young males aged between 25 and 45 with no known history of metabolic or cardiovascular diseases. Abdominal obesity was defined based on the International Diabetes Federation (IDF) criteria, i.e., WC ≥ 94 cm [38], and obesity was defined as BMI ≥ 30 kg/m^2. The mean BMI in hookah smokers was significantly higher than that of nonsmokers (28.2 ± 3.6 vs. 26.5 ± 2.6; $p = 0.046$), and there was a higher prevalence of obesity (37.9% vs. 6.9%; $p = 0.04$) and a higher prevalence of abdominal obesity (79.3% vs. 59.6%; $p = 0.08$) among hookah smokers.

3.2. Meta-Analysis

The meta-analysis results estimating the overall risk ratios for obesity in hookah smokers compared to nonsmokers are presented in Figure 2. The random effect weighted pooled risk for obesity in hookah smokers indicated an increased risk of obesity of approximately 38%, compared to nonsmokers (RR = 1.38; 95% CI = 1.02–1.87; $p = 0.04$). The heterogeneity analysis revealed a moderate variability ($I^2 = 53\%$).

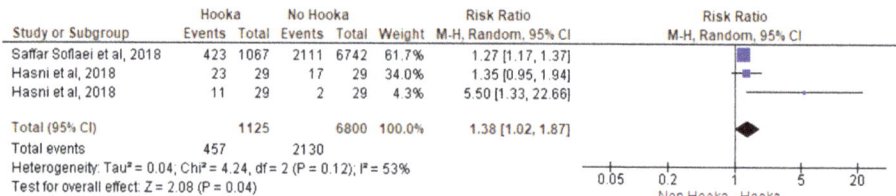

Figure 2. The forest plot for the risk of obesity with hookah-smoking.

4. Discussion

The aim of the current systematic review was to provide benchmark data on the association between hookah smoking and obesity. Five studies, comprising a total of 16,779 adolescent and adult participants and age range between 13–75 years and conducted in Iran, Syria, Jordan, Pakistan, and Tunisia, met the inclusion criteria and were reviewed, revealing one major finding: All five studies included in our systematic review showed a higher prevalence of obesity and/or a higher association between obesity (abdominal obesity, BMI percentile ≥ 95th, or BMI ≥ 30 kg/m^2) and hookah smoking than the corresponding values for nonsmokers and cigarette smokers (when comparisons were available) regardless of gender and among all ages. This finding is considered to be strong and robust because (i) data were derived from well-conducted, large-sample, population-based studies with a low risk of bias; (ii) the finding was not contradicted in any of the included studies; (iii) the same finding has also been reported in clinical samples (i.e., not the general population) [39]; and (iv) this finding was confirmed by a meta-analysis.

4.1. Clinical Implications

Our findings have some implications, especially for the general population. Firstly, it is important to discuss the association between hookah smoking and obesity among young adults, perhaps through educational interventions in schools and universities and in work settings [40,41]. In addition, the common public belief that hookah smoking may be healthy, since hookah smoke contains fruit flavours and the water in the bottom of the hookah can eliminate the toxicity of tobacco compared with cigarettes, should be contradicted. On the contrary, we found that the adverse effects of hookah smoking could be even greater than those of cigarette smoking. In fact, several types of cancer (e.g., lung cancer) have been linked to hookah smoking [42]. Moreover, it causes coronary artery disease [39], an increased heart rate and high blood pressure [43], respiratory diseases [10], dental problems [44], and osteoporosis [45], as well as infections when sharing a hookah [45].

It is unclear why smoking hookah is associated with obesity; we speculate that the potential mechanisms behind this association may be multiple. However, two factors may have a major impact. Firstly, smoking a hookah requires sitting, and a hookah-smoking session may last for two hours. Some individuals may repeat the session two or three times a day [46], and this unavoidably facilitates a sedentary lifestyle (unlike cigarettes), which reduces energy expenditure [47]. Also, the hookah is smoked during social events where smokers spend time together and talk as they pass the mouthpiece around in environments (e.g., restaurants and coffee shops) rich in eating stimuli, which could increase the exposure to and consumption of high-calorie foods [47]. All in all, it has been shown that hookah smoking is associated with less healthy lifestyle habits in both men and women [48].

4.2. Strengths and Limitations

This systematic review has certain strengths. To the best of our knowledge, this is the first systematic review to investigate the association between hookah smoking and obesity. Despite the fact that few studies met the inclusion criteria and were included in our systematic review, the finding is considered to be strong, with definite evidence for the association between hookah smoking and obesity. This needs to be underlined due to the increasing trend of this smoking habit, especially

J. Cardiovasc. Dev. Dis. **2019**, *6*, 23

among young people. However, this systematic review also has certain limitations. In particular, our results should be interpreted with caution with regard to the association between hookah smoking and obesity, since the cross-sectional design of the studies included in our systematic review indicates only simple associations at best and does not provide solid information regarding any causal relationships between conditions [49]. In other words, these studies lack evidence to determine whether hookah smoking may lead to obesity, since very few studies have longitudinally investigated the "real" effects of hookah smoking [50]. Moreover, the included studies in our systematic review were conducted only in low-middle income countries (i.e., Middle East); therefore, our findings may not be generalized on a global scale. Finally, none of the included studies clearly examined if the average number of sessions (i.e., per day or week) or years (i.e., months and years) of hookah smoking are related to a higher risk of obesity. All these shortcomings in the current research indicate the need to design longitudinal studies to clarify the real effect of hookah smoking on the onset and progression of obesity and weight-related comorbidities, especially in Western countries (i.e., US and Europe).

5. Conclusions

Despite the scarcity of studies, the preliminary findings indicate a high prevalence of obesity in hookah smokers. Public health policymakers should be aware of this for the better management of obesity and other diseases related to hookah smoking.

Author Contributions: All authors claim authorship to, have approved of, and made substantial contribution to the conception, drafting, and final version of the paper.

Funding: The authors received no funding.

Conflicts of Interest: The authors declare no conflict of interest.

References

1. Ray, C. The hookah—The Indian waterpipe. *Curr. Sci.* **2009**, *96*, 1319–1323.
2. Brockman, L.N.; Pumper, M.A.; Christakis, D.A.; Moreno, M.A. Hookah's new popularity among US college students: A pilot study of the characteristics of hookah smokers and their Facebook displays. *BMJ Open* **2012**, *2*, e001709. [CrossRef] [PubMed]
3. Maziak, W.; Taleb, Z.B.; Bahelah, R.; Islam, F.; Jaber, R.; Auf, R.; Salloum, R.G. The global epidemiology of waterpipe smoking. *Tob. Control* **2015**, *24*, i3–i12. [CrossRef] [PubMed]
4. Soule, E.K.; Lipato, T.; Eissenberg, T. Waterpipe tobacco smoking: A new smoking epidemic among the young? *Curr. Pulmonol. Rep.* **2015**, *4*, 163–172. [CrossRef]
5. Szyfter, A.; Giefing, M. Is waterpipe smoking a safe alterative for cigarette smoking? *Przegl. Lek.* **2012**, *69*, 1090–1094. [PubMed]
6. Awan, K.H.; Siddiqi, K.; Patil, S.; Hussain, Q.A. Assessing the Effect of Waterpipe Smoking on Cancer Outcome—A Systematic Review of Current Evidence. *Asian Pac. J. Cancer Prev.* **2017**, *18*, 495–502.
7. Lai, H.T.; Koriyama, C.; Tokudome, S.; Tran, H.H.; Tran, L.T.; Nandakumar, A.; Akiba, S.; Le, N.T. Waterpipe Tobacco Smoking and Gastric Cancer Risk among Vietnamese Men. *PLoS ONE* **2016**, *11*, e0165587. [CrossRef] [PubMed]
8. Montazeri, Z.; Nyiraneza, C.; El-Katerji, H.; Little, J. Waterpipe smoking and cancer: Systematic review and meta-analysis. *Tob. Control* **2017**, *26*, 92–97. [CrossRef]
9. Warnakulasuriya, S. Waterpipe smoking, oral cancer and other oral health effects. *Evid. Based Dent.* **2011**, *12*, 44–45. [CrossRef]
10. Meo, S.A.; AlShehri, K.A.; AlHarbi, B.B.; Barayyan, O.R.; Bawazir, A.S.; Alanazi, O.A.; Al-Zuhair, A.R. Effect of shisha (waterpipe) smoking on lung functions and fractional exhaled nitric oxide (FeNO) among Saudi young adult shisha smokers. *Int. J. Environ. Res. Public Health* **2014**, *11*, 9638–9648. [CrossRef]
11. Bahtouee, M.; Maleki, N.; Nekouee, F. The prevalence of chronic obstructive pulmonary disease in hookah smokers. *Chron. Respir. Dis.* **2018**, *15*, 165–172. [CrossRef] [PubMed]
12. She, J.; Yang, P.; Wang, Y.; Qin, X.; Fan, J.; Wang, Y.; Gao, G.; Luo, G.; Ma, K.; Li, B.; et al. Chinese water-pipe smoking and the risk of COPD. *Chest* **2014**, *146*, 924–931. [CrossRef] [PubMed]

13. Aslam, H.M.; Saleem, S.; German, S.; Qureshi, W.A. Harmful effects of shisha: Literature review. *Int. Arch. Med.* **2014**, *7*, 16. [CrossRef] [PubMed]
14. Nelson, M.D.; Rezk-Hanna, M.; Rader, F.; Mason, O.R.; Tang, X.; Shidban, S.; Rosenberry, R.; Benowitz, N.L.; Tashkin, D.P.; Elashoff, R.M.; et al. Acute Effect of Hookah Smoking on the Human Coronary Microcirculation. *Am. J. Cardiol.* **2016**, *117*, 1747–1754. [CrossRef] [PubMed]
15. Bhatnagar, A.; Maziak, W.; Eissenberg, T.; Ward, K.D.; Thurston, G.; King, B.A.; Sutfin, E.L.; Cobb, C.O.; Griffiths, M.; Goldstein, L.B.; et al. Water Pipe (Hookah) Smoking and Cardiovascular Disease Risk: A Scientific Statement from the American Heart Association. *Circulation* **2019**, *139*, e917–e936. [CrossRef] [PubMed]
16. El Ghoch, M.; Fakhoury, R. Challenges and New Directions in Obesity Management: Lifestyle modification programs, pharmacotherapy and Bariatric surgery. *J. Popul. Ther. Clin. Pharmacol.* **2019**, *26*, e1–e4.
17. Kreidieh, D.; Itani, L.; El Masri, D.; Tannir, H.; Citarella, R.; El Ghoch, M. Association between Sarcopenic Obesity, Type 2 Diabetes, and Hypertension in Overweight and Obese Treatment-Seeking Adult Women. *J. Cardiovasc. Dev. Dis.* **2018**, *5*, 51. [CrossRef]
18. Khazem, S.; Itani, L.; Kreidieh, D.; El Masri, D.; Tannir, H.; Citarella, R.; El Ghoch, M. Reduced Lean Body Mass and Cardiometabolic Diseases in Adult Males with Overweight and Obesity: A Pilot Study. *Int. J. Environ. Res. Public Health* **2018**, *15*, 2754. [CrossRef]
19. Kreidieh, D.; Itani, L.; El Kassas, G.; El Masri, D.; Calugi, S.; Grave, R.D.; El Ghoch, M. Long-term Lifestyle-modification Programs for Overweight and Obesity Management in the Arab States: Systematic Review and Meta-analysis. *Curr. Diabetes Rev.* **2018**, *14*, 550–558. [CrossRef]
20. Itani, L.; Calugi, S.; Dalle Grave, R.; Kreidieh, D.; El Kassas, G.; El Masri, D.; Tannir, H.; Harfoush, A.; El Ghoch, M. The Association between Body Mass Index and Health-Related Quality of Life in Treatment-Seeking Arab Adults with Obesity. *Med. Sci.* **2018**, *6*, 25. [CrossRef]
21. Rodgers, J.L.; Jones, J.; Bolleddu, S.I.; Vanthenapalli, S.; Rodgers, L.E.; Shah, K.; Karia, K.; Panguluri, S.K. Cardiovascular Risks Associated with Gender and Aging. *J. Cardiovasc. Dev. Dis.* **2019**, *6*, 19. [CrossRef] [PubMed]
22. Lowe, Y. *Smoking Shisha Linked to Diabetes and Obesity, Study Finds*; The Telegraph: London, UK, 2019.
23. Richardson, W.S.; Wilson, M.C.; Nishikawa, J.; Hayward, R.S. The well-built clinical question: A key to evidence-based decisions. *ACP J. Club* **1995**, *123*, A12–A13. [PubMed]
24. Sawyer, S.M.; Azzopardi, P.S.; Wickremarathne, D.; Patton, G.C. The age of adolescence. *Lancet Child Adolesc. Health* **2018**, *2*, 223–228. [CrossRef]
25. Liberati, A.; Altman, D.G.; Tetzlaff, J.; Mulrow, C.; Gotzsche, P.C.; Ioannidis, J.P.; Clarke, M.; Devereaux, P.J.; Kleijnen, J.; Moher, D. The PRISMA statement for reporting systematic reviews and meta-analyses of studies that evaluate health care interventions: Explanation and elaboration. *Ann. Int. Med.* **2009**, *151*, W65–W94. [CrossRef] [PubMed]
26. Liberati, A.; Altman, D.G.; Tetzlaff, J.; Mulrow, C.; Gotzsche, P.C.; Ioannidis, J.P.; Clarke, M.; Devereaux, P.J.; Kleijnen, J.; Moher, D. The PRISMA statement for reporting systematic reviews and meta-analyses of studies that evaluate health care interventions: Explanation and elaboration. *PLOS Med.* **2009**, *6*. [CrossRef] [PubMed]
27. Davies, S. The importance of PROSPERO to the National Institute for Health Research. *Syst Rev.* **2012**, *1*, 5. [CrossRef]
28. Hoy, D.; Brooks, P.; Woolf, A.; Blyth, F.; March, L.; Bain, C.; Baker, P.; Smith, E.; Buchbinder, R. Assessing risk of bias in prevalence studies: Modification of an existing tool and evidence of interrater agreement. *J. Clin. Epidemiol.* **2012**, *65*, 934–939. [CrossRef]
29. Popay, J.; Roberts, H.; Sowden, A.; Petticrew, M.; Britten, N.; Arai, L.; Rodgers, M.; Britten, N.; Roen, K.; Duffy, S. Developing guidance on the conduct of narrative synthesis in systematic reviews. *J. Epidemiol. Community Health* **2005**, *59*, A7.
30. Campbell, M.; Katikireddi, S.V.; Sowden, A.; Thomson, H. Lack of transparency in reporting narrative synthesis of quantitative data: A methodological assessment of systematic reviews. *J. Clin. Epidemiol.* **2019**, *105*, 1–9. [CrossRef]
31. *Review Manager (RevMan)*; Version 5.3; The Nordic Cochrane Centre: Copenhagen, Denmark; The Cochrane: London, UK, 2014.

J. Cardiovasc. Dev. Dis. **2019**, *6*, 23

32. Shafique, K.; Mirza, S.S.; Mughal, M.K.; Arain, Z.I.; Khan, N.A.; Tareen, M.F.; Ahmad, I. Water-pipe smoking and metabolic syndrome: A population-based study. *PLoS ONE* **2012**, *7*, e39734. [CrossRef]

33. Misra, A.; Vikram, N.K.; Gupta, R.; Pandey, R.M.; Wasir, J.S.; Gupta, V.P. Waist circumference cutoff points and action levels for Asian Indians for identification of abdominal obesity. *Int. J. Obes.* **2006**, *30*, 106–111. [CrossRef] [PubMed]

34. Ward, K.D.; Ahn, S.; Mzayek, F.; Al Ali, R.; Rastam, S.; Asfar, T.; Fouad, F.; Maziak, W. The relationship between waterpipe smoking and body weight: Population-based findings from Syria. *Nicotine Tob. Res.* **2015**, *17*, 34–40. [CrossRef] [PubMed]

35. Saffar Soflaei, S.; Darroudi, S.; Tayefi, M.; Nosrati Tirkani, A.; Moohebati, M.; Ebrahimi, M.; Esmaily, H.; Parizadeh, S.M.R.; Heidari-Bakavoli, A.R.; Ferns, G.A.; et al. Hookah smoking is strongly associated with diabetes mellitus, metabolic syndrome and obesity: A population-based study. *Diabetol. Metab. Syndr.* **2018**, *10*, 33. [CrossRef]

36. Alomari, M.A.; Al-Sheyab, N.A.; Ward, K.D. Adolescent Waterpipe Use is Associated with Greater Body Weight: The Irbid-TRY. *Subst. Use Misuse* **2018**, *53*, 1194–1202. [CrossRef]

37. Hasni, Y.; Bachrouch, S.; Mahjoub, M.; Maaroufi, A.; Rouatbi, S.; Ben Saad, H. Biochemical Data and Metabolic Profiles of Male Exclusive Narghile Smokers (ENSs) Compared with Apparently Healthy Nonsmokers (AHNSs). *Am. J. Men's Health* **2019**, *13*. [CrossRef]

38. Alberti, K.G.; Zimmet, P.; Shaw, J. Metabolic syndrome—A new world-wide definition. A Consensus Statement from the International Diabetes Federation. *Diabet. Med.* **2006**, *23*, 469–480. [CrossRef] [PubMed]

39. Selim, G.M.; Fouad, H.; Ezzat, S. Impact of shisha smoking on the extent of coronary artery disease in patients referred for coronary angiography. *Anadolu Kardiyol Derg* **2013**, *13*, 647–654. [CrossRef] [PubMed]

40. Campbell, R.; Starkey, F.; Holliday, J.; Audrey, S.; Bloor, M.; Parry-Langdon, N.; Hughes, R.; Moore, L. An informal school-based peer-led intervention for smoking prevention in adolescence (ASSIST): A cluster randomised trial. *Lancet* **2008**, *371*, 1595–1602. [CrossRef]

41. Brown, J.; Michie, S.; Geraghty, A.W.; Yardley, L.; Gardner, B.; Shahab, L.; Stapleton, J.A.; West, R. Internet-based intervention for smoking cessation (StopAdvisor) in people with low and high socioeconomic status: A randomised controlled trial. *Lancet Respir. Med.* **2014**, *2*, 997–1006. [CrossRef]

42. Koul, P.A.; Hajni, M.R.; Sheikh, M.A.; Khan, U.H.; Shah, A.; Khan, Y.; Ahangar, A.G.; Tasleem, R.A. Hookah smoking and lung cancer in the Kashmir valley of the Indian subcontinent. *Asian Pac. J. Cancer Prev.* **2011**, *12*, 519–524. [PubMed]

43. Kadhum, M.; Jaffery, A.; Haq, A.; Bacon, J.; Madden, B. Measuring the acute cardiovascular effects of shisha smoking: A cross-sectional study. *JRSM Open* **2014**, *5*. [CrossRef] [PubMed]

44. Kasat, V.; Ladda, R. Smoking and dental implants. *J. Int. Soc. Prev. Commun. Dent.* **2012**, *2*, 38–41. [CrossRef] [PubMed]

45. El-Zaatari, Z.M.; Chami, H.A.; Zaatari, G.S. Health effects associated with waterpipe smoking. *Tob. Control* **2015**, *24*, i31–i43. [CrossRef] [PubMed]

46. Robinson, J.N.; Wang, B.; Jackson, K.J.; Donaldson, E.A.; Ryant, C.A. Characteristics of Hookah Tobacco Smoking Sessions and Correlates of Use Frequency Among US Adults: Findings from Wave 1 of the Population Assessment of Tobacco and Health (PATH) Study. *Nicotine Tob. Res.* **2018**, *20*, 731–740. [CrossRef] [PubMed]

47. Momenabadi, V.; Hossein Kaveh Ph, D.M.; Hashemi, S.Y.; Borhaninejad, V.R. Factors Affecting Hookah Smoking Trend in the Society: A Review Article. *Addict. Health* **2016**, *8*, 123–135. [PubMed]

48. Abdollahifard, G.; Vakili, V.; Danaei, M.; Askarian, M.; Romito, L.; Palenik, C.J. Are the Predictors of Hookah Smoking Differ from Those of Cigarette Smoking? Report of a population-based study in Shiraz, Iran, 2010. *Int. J. Prev. Med.* **2013**, *4*, 459–466.

49. Solem, R.C. Limitation of a cross-sectional study. *Am. J. Orthod. Dentofac. Orthop.* **2015**, *148*, 205. [CrossRef]

50. Caruana, E.J.; Roman, M.; Hernandez-Sanchez, J.; Solli, P. Longitudinal studies. *J. Thorac. Dis.* **2015**, *7*, E537–E540.

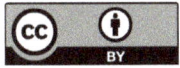

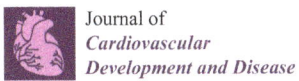
Journal of
Cardiovascular
Development and Disease

MDPI

Review

An Update on the Tissue Renin Angiotensin System and Its Role in Physiology and Pathology

Ali Nehme [1], Fouad A. Zouein [2], Zeinab Deris Zayeri [3] and Kazem Zibara [4,*]

[1] EA4173, Functional genomics of arterial hypertension, Univeristy Claude Bernard Lyon-1 (UCBL-1), 69008 Lyon, France; ali.hassan.nehme@gmail.com
[2] Department of Pharmacology and Toxicology, Heart Repair Division, Faculty of Medicine, American University of Beirut, Beirut 11-0236, Lebanon; fz15@aub.edu.lb
[3] Thalassemia & Hemoglobinopathy Research Center, Health Research Institute, Ahvaz Jundishapur University of Medical Sciences, Ahvaz, Iran; zeynabderisgenetice@gmail.com
[4] PRASE, Biology Department, Faculty of Sciences-I, Lebanese University, Beirut, Lebanon
* Correspondence: kzibara@ul.edu.lb

Received: 10 February 2019; Accepted: 26 March 2019; Published: 29 March 2019

Abstract: In its classical view, the renin angiotensin system (RAS) was defined as an endocrine system involved in blood pressure regulation and body electrolyte balance. However, the emerging concept of tissue RAS, along with the discovery of new RAS components, increased the physiological and clinical relevance of the system. Indeed, RAS has been shown to be expressed in various tissues where alterations in its expression were shown to be involved in multiple diseases including atherosclerosis, cardiac hypertrophy, type 2 diabetes (T2D) and renal fibrosis. In this chapter, we describe the new components of RAS, their tissue-specific expression, and their alterations under pathological conditions, which will help achieve more tissue- and condition-specific treatments.

Keywords: renin-angiotensin-aldosterone system; tissue; expression; physiology

1. Introduction

In its classical view, RAS was defined as an endocrine system involved in blood pressure regulation and body electrolyte balance. However, RAS is now considered a "ubiquitous" system that is expressed locally in various tissues and exerts multiple paracrine/autocrine effects involved in tissue physiology and homeostasis [1]. Indeed, RAS plays key roles in cellular growth, proliferation, differentiation, migration, and apoptosis, in addition to extracellular matrix (ECM) remodeling and inflammation [2].

Alterations in RAS expression were shown to be involved in multiple diseases including atherosclerosis, cardiac hypertrophy, type 2 diabetes, and renal fibrosis [2–4]. On the other hand, RAS-blocking agents, such as angiotensin converting enzyme (ACE) inhibitors and AT1 receptor blockers (ARBs), have been shown to be effective in the management of hypertension-related cardiovascular diseases and end-organ damage [5]. Therefore, it is necessary to know the components of RAS, their tissue-specific expression, and how they may change under pathological conditions. In this review, we discuss classical and novel components of RAS, their role in local tissue physiology, and their changes under specific pathological conditions. A better understanding of local tissue RAS expression and regulation will help achieve more tissue- and condition-specific treatments.

2. An Overview of RAS

In its classical view, RAS includes successive enzymatic reactions resulting in the conversion of the "inactive" substrate angiotensinogen (AGT), into the active peptide angiotensin II (Ang-II) which binds to its specific membrane receptors and elicits cellular effects [2] (Figure 1 and Table 1). AGT is a glycoprotein continuously produced by the liver. In addition, it is differentially expressed in multiple other tissues, including heart, blood vessels, kidneys, and adipose tissue [2]. AGT production can be induced by several stimuli, including inflammation, insulin, estrogen, glucocorticoids, thyroid hormone, and Ang-II [6].

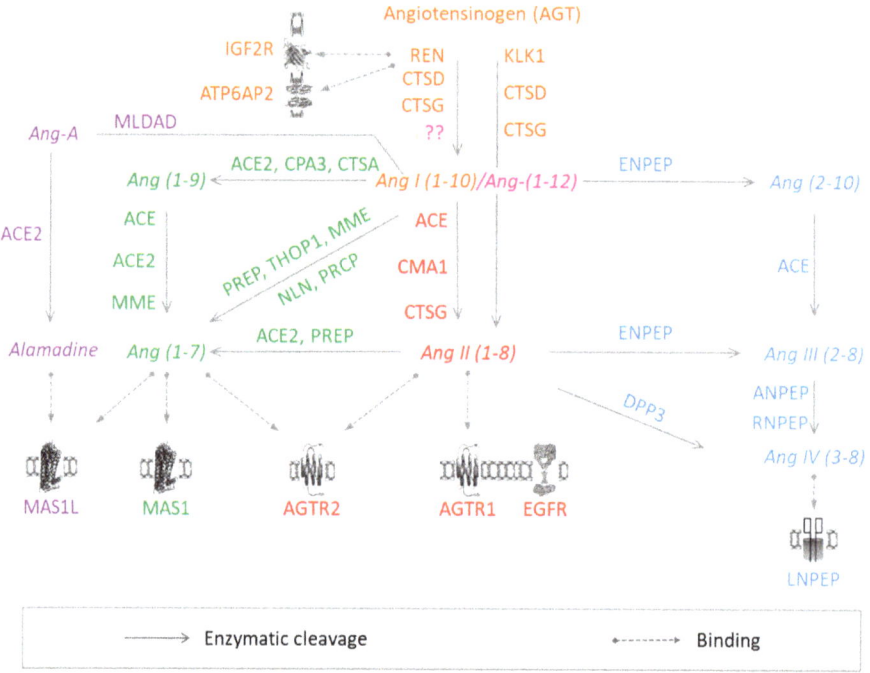

Figure 1. RAS components. Colors correspond to different arms of RAS: Orange, Angiotensin-I; pink, Angiotensin-(1–12); red, Angiotensin-II; green, Angiotensin-(1–7); Blue, Angiotensin III/VI; violet, Alamandine. Proteins are represented by the corresponding official gene symbols. The figure was adapted from Nehme et al. 2015 [7].

In the plasma, AGT is converted into the decapeptide angiotensin-I (1–10) (Ang-I) by renin (Figure 1 and Table 1), a tightly regulated enzyme produced by the juxtaglomerular cells (JG) [8]. In fact, this step is considered the rate limiting step of Ang-II release in the circulation [8]. Renin is synthesized as an inactive enzyme that is cleaved by microsomes to produce prorenin [9]. Prorenin is then either released as inactive precursor or converted by a variety of proteases into active intracellular renin that is stored in granules of the JG cells. Active renin is released into the circulation by JG cells via an exocytic process and upon a stimulus [8,10] by different mechanisms including Ang-II negative feedback [10].

Ang-I is further processed by angiotensin-converting enzyme (ACE), a membrane-bound exopeptidase, to release the vasoactive octapeptide angiotensin II (1–8) (Ang-II) (Figure 1 and Table 1). Besides Ang-II production, ACE can degrade a number of vasodilating peptides including Ang-(1–7), bradykinin, and kallikrein, thus playing a central role as a vasopressor enzyme [2,8]. Moreover, ACE can activate cellular signaling when bound to its inhibitors (ACEIs) and bradykinin, leading to increased ACE and COX2 production [11].

Table 1. Extended renin-angiotensin-aldosterone system components.

Gene Symbol	Gene Description	Gene ID
ACE *	angiotensin I converting enzyme (peptidyl-dipeptidase A) 1	1636
ACE2	angiotensin I converting enzyme (peptidyl-dipeptidase A) 2	59272
AGT *	angiotensinogen (serpin peptidase inhibitor, clade A, member 8)	183
AGTR1 *	angiotensin II receptor, type 1	185
AGTR2	angiotensin II receptor, type 2	186
ANPEP	alanyl (membrane) aminopeptidase	290
ATP6AP2	ATPase, H+ transporting, lysosomal accessory protein 2	10159
CMA1	chymase 1, mast cell	1215
CPA3	carboxypeptidase A3 (mast cell)	1359
CTSA	cathepsin A	5476
CTSD	cathepsin D	1509
CTSG	cathepsin G	1511
DPP3	dipeptidyl-peptidase 3	10072
EGFR	epidermal growth factor receptor	1956
ENPEP	glutamyl aminopeptidase (aminopeptidase A)	2028
IGF2R	insulin-like growth factor 2 receptor	3482
KLK1	kallikrein 1	3816
LNPEP	leucyl/cystinyl aminopeptidase	4012
MAS1	MAS1 oncogene	4142
MME	membrane metallo-endopeptidase	4311
NLN	neurolysin (metallopeptidase M3 family)	57486
PREP	prolyl endopeptidase	5550
REN *	renin	5972
RNPEP	arginyl aminopeptidase (aminopeptidase B)	6051
THOP1	thimet oligopeptidase 1	7064
AKR1C4	aldo-keto reductase family 1, member C4	1109
AKR1D1	aldo-keto reductase family 1, member D1	6718
CYP11A1	cytochrome P450, family 11, subfamily A, polypeptide 1	1583
CYP11B1	cytochrome P450, family 11, subfamily B, polypeptide 1	1584
CYP11B2 *	cytochrome P450, family 11, subfamily B, polypeptide 2	1585
CYP17A1	cytochrome P450, family 17, subfamily A, polypeptide 1	1586
CYP21A2	cytochrome P450, family 21, subfamily A, polypeptide 2	1589
GPER	G protein-coupled estrogen receptor 1	2852
HSD11B1	hydroxysteroid (11-beta) dehydrogenase 1	3290
HSD11B2 *	hydroxysteroid (11-beta) dehydrogenase 2	3291
NR3C1	nuclear receptor subfamily 3, group C, member 1 (glucocorticoid receptor)	2908
NR3C2 *	nuclear receptor subfamily 3, group C, member 2 (Mineralocorticoid receptor)	4306

* Classical RAS components.

Ang-II is a biologically active peptide that mediates its effects via the angiotensin-II type 1 receptor (AT1R) [12] (Figure 1). Ang-II was originally known as a circulating hormone that regulates blood pressure and electrolyte balance by acting on vascular contraction, aldosterone secretion, renal sodium handling, sympathetic activity, and vasopressin release [2]. However, molecular studies have shown that AT1R activation can exert long-term genetic effects, in addition to rapid short term effects at the cellular level [13]. Like most other GPCRs, AT1R undergoes rapid desensitization and internalization after agonist stimulation to avoid extensive chronic activation [2].

One of the major effects of Ang-II is the stimulation of aldosterone synthase, CYP11B2, expression in the adrenal cortex [14] (Figure 1 and Table 1). Aldosterone has emerged as an essential regulator of blood pressure in mammals, and has been associated with a variety of diseases in humans [15]. Aldosterone acts in a variety of tissues through its mineralocorticoid receptor (MR) to influence extracellular fluid volume, blood pressure and salt exchange, but may also lead to pathological consequences, mainly tissue fibrosis and oxidative stress [16].

3. The Concept of Tissue RAS

Several lines of evidence support the concept of extended RAS that includes multiple synonymous enzymatic pathways for the generation of different angiotensin peptides which exert their effects in a tissue- and condition-specific manner [17]. These pathways may explain the dual role of RAS as not only a circulating hormone, but also a tissue-specific regulatory system serving autocrine, paracrine, and even intracrine functions.

The first demonstration of the presence of a local tissue RAS was in 1971, where a renin-like activity was found in the brain of dogs and which was independent of renin found in the kidney and plasma [18]. This finding was then supported by the identification of Ang-I-like peptides in dog brain with variable molecular weights [19]. Since then, local angiotensin pathways and their physiological importance were elucidated in different tissues including the heart, blood vessels, kidney, brain, adipose tissue, adrenal gland, pancreas, liver, reproductive system, lymphatic tissue, placenta and the eye (Table 2) [2,20,21]. In these tissues, local RAS acts independently from systemic RAS in a paracrine and autocrine manner, but may still interact with systemic RAS to exert endocrine effects [2]. A study conducted by Lau et al. showed a local angiotensin-generating system in the exocrine pancreas. Their data showed the existence of an islet angiotensin-generating system that has an important role in physiological regulation of glucose-induced insulin secretion [22]. In addition, recent studies have reported the expression of renin and angiotensinogen genes and identified their products at many local tissue sites, which further supports the concept of multiple tissues synthesizing RAS components [23]. In fact, multiple studies have described tissue RAS and reported its role in various tissues such as cardiac, vascular and renal tissues, which have the majority of ACE in the body. It seems that tissue RAS has long-term effects on cardiovascular function and structure, while its alteration can cause pathologic conditions [24].

Table 2. The physiological and pathophysiological role of RAS in different tissues.

Tissue	Physiological Role of RAS	Associated Diseases
Blood vessel	Vasomotor regulation, oxidative metabolism	Hypertension, atherosclerosis
Heart	Vasomotor tone, fibrotic regulation, oxidative metabolism	Heart failure, cardiac hypertrophy and fibrosis
Kidney	Blood pressure regulation	Chronic kidney disease
CNS	Sympathetic regulation of blood pressure	Hypertension
Adipose tissue	Adipogenesis	Insulin resistance and obesity
Eye	Aqueous humor dynamics	Glaucoma and diabetic retinopathy
Liver	Glucose metabolism	Glucose intolerance and fibrosis

3.1. Angiotensin-I

Apart from Renin, several enzymes were found to cleave angiotensinogen into Ang-I, such as cathepsin D (CTSD), cathepsin G (CTSG), and tonins [25] (Figure 1). In addition, studies have shown that three main receptors can be bound and activated by renin, which are: renin-binding protein (RnBP), mannose 6-phosphate/insulin-like growth factor II (M6P/IGFII) receptor and the renin/prorenin receptor (R/PR) [26] (Figure 1 and Table 1). Although RnBP is known to be a renin inhibitor, the latter two are known to increase renin catalytic activity and activate intracellular signaling [20]. R/PR binding is supposed to induce full non-proteolytic activation of prorenin by a conformational change, through which prorenin active site is exposed [26]. The interaction between R/PR and prorenin is species-specific, which may explain the lack of rat prorenin activation by human R/PR [27].

The concept of local RAS was initially challenged by the fact that renin was considered the rate-limiting specific enzyme to cleave AGT into Ang-I [28]. However, renin mRNA and/or activity was detected in several extra-renal tissues, including the vascular wall [29], cardiac [30], adipose [31], and eye tissues [32]. In addition, M6P/IGFII receptor, encoded by the IGF2R gene, contribute to the uptake and activation of M6P-containing prorenin from the circulation at different tissues and in a variety of cells including cardiomyocytes [33], fibroblasts, VSMCs, and ECs [26,33]. On the other hand, the P/PR was shown to be expressed and active in diverse tissues, including the kidney, vascular wall, brain, and the eye. Alterations in R/PR are associated with pathologies such as glomerulosclerosis, diabetes, hypertension, neovascularization and inflammation [26].

In fact, renin is considered the rate limiting enzyme for the generation of Ang-I in plasma, whereas in tissues, enzymes other than renin are thought to regulate Ang-I generation [34]. Of importance is CTSD, which is a ubiquitous lysosomal aspartyl protease [35] that was shown to provide an alternative angiotensin production pathway after myocardial infarction, and hence falsely increase clinical plasma renin activity determinations [36]. Cathepsin D knockdown by siRNA led to more than a two-fold reduction in intracellular and extracellular Ang-I and Ang-II production by VSMCs under both normal and high glucose concentrations [37]. Interestingly, however, silencing of tissue plasminogen activator (tPA) gene, previously associated with Ang-II production [38], moderately increased intracellular Ang-I and Ang-II levels in VSMCs only under high glucose concentrations, while strongly decreased Ang-I and Ang-II levels in the media [37]. However, a consensus on the renin-compensatory activity of CTSD has not been reached yet due to the low specificity and efficiency of CTSD, which has been found to only metabolize AGT under acidic conditions [39,40].

Despite the importance of this rate limiting step in RAS, little effort has been made to further support local Ang-I generation from renin or renin-like enzymes. Therefore, further studies should be performed to identify local mechanisms involved in angiotensinogen cleavage, either through renin recruitment from the circulation, or through local renin-independent enzymatic reactions.

3.2. Angiotensin (1–12)

One of the recent important discoveries in RAS is the identification of the Angiotensin (1–12) peptide (Ang-(1–12)), which may serve as an alternative precursor for the production of bioactive angiotensin peptides, independent from Ang-I production [41]. Ang-(1–12) was first isolated by Nagata et al. from rat small intestine, and was shown to induce constriction of aortic strips ex vivo and to raise blood pressure in rats when infused intravenously [41]. Both the vasoconstrictor and pressor responses to Ang-(1–12) were abolished by ACE inhibitors (ACEI) and AT1R blockers (ARBs), which suggest a renin-independent pathway for angiotensin peptides production [41,42]. Despite the differences in amino acid sequence of rat and human Ang-(1–12), Ferrario et al. showed cardiac production of Ang-(1–12) in a rat model expressing human AGT [43].

In addition, compelling evidence suggests that Ang-(1–12) is a major source for local Ang-II production in the central nervous system. Endogenous neutralization of Ang-(1–12) using antibodies directed against the C-terminal end of Ang-(1–12) into a lateral cerebral ventricle of (mRen2)27 transgenic hypertensive rats prompted blood pressure reduction that was associated with a transient anti-dipsogenic behavior [44]. Central effects of Ang-(1–12) were later shown to be mediated via the Ang-II/AT1R axis in the solitary tract nucleus and hypothalamic arcuate nucleus [45–47]. Ang-(1–12) was also shown to be present abundantly in a wide range of rat organs and tissues, including heart ventricular myocytes, small intestine, spleen, kidneys, and liver [41]. Lower levels were also found in the medial layer of intracoronary arteries and vascular endothelium [48]. Despite the increase in plasma renin activity following low-salt feeding, the levels of Ang-I, Ang-II, and Ang-(1–12) in plasma and various tissues remained unchanged [49], which suggests that Ang-(1–12) metabolism is regulated in a manner that is independent of circulating renin activity.

Studies on Ang-(1–12) clearly demonstrate species-specific, tissue-specific, and condition-specific metabolism that favors one pathway or enzyme, over the others [17]. For instance, Jessup et al.

showed that Ang-(1–12) immunoreactivity was detected in both the heart and kidney of spontaneously hypertensive rats (SHR) and Wistar–Kyoto (WKY) rats. However, tissue measurements by radioimmunoassay showed higher cardiac and lower renal levels of Ang-(1–12) in SHR, compared with WKY rats [48]. It was shown that Ang-(1–12) was cleaved by ACE to generate both Ang-I and Ang-II in rat serum, independent of renin participation [50]. On the other hand, the same team showed that Ang-(1–7) and Ang-(1–4) were the main products of Ang-(1–12) metabolism in renal cortical membranes of rats, which were abolished by neprilysin inhibition [50]. In addition, myocytes of WKY rats were shown to sequester Ang-(1–12) in culture, which was mainly metabolized by ACE and membrane metallo-endopeptidase (MME) [51]. Interestingly, the uptake and metabolism were higher in cardiomyocytes obtained from SHR rats with a predominant effect of chymase in these cells [52]. On the other hand, chymase was shown to be the major enzyme contributing to Ang-(1–12) cleavage in an isolated heart model of cardiac ischaemia-reperfusion injury in Sprague–Dawley rats [53]. ACEI, however, but not chymostatin, inhibited circulatory Ang-(1–12) production in both SHR and WKY rats[42].

Ang-(1–12) production and metabolism have raised concerns about the possible role of this peptide in mitigating the effects of renin and ACE inhibitors in the treatment of heart failure, which warrant further studies to identify tissue-specific RAS metabolic targets for disease treatment.

3.3. Angiotensin-II

In addition to the ACE-dependent cleavage of Ang-I, Ang-II can also be produced by the direct cleavage of AGT by cathepsin G [54], tonin, and kallikrein, or through Ang-I cleavage by chymase and cathepsin G[216] (Figure 1 and Table 1). Of importance, chymase, a serine protease that is highly specific to the Phe^8-His^9 bond [17] of Ang-I, was shown to be more active than ACE in generating Ang-II in human heart [55] and diabetic kidneys [56].

In addition to AT1R (Figure 1 and Table 1), Ang-II also acts through AT2R, a seven transmembrane receptor that acts mainly through Gi and tyrosine phosphatases to exert inhibitory actions on cellular responses mediated by AT1R, mainly by inhibiting cell growth and proliferation while promoting cell differentiation, in addition to vasodilation and reducing blood pressure [57].

Ang-II was thought for a long time to be only a circulating peptide, exerting its effects through endocrine mechanisms. However, many studies identified Ang-II in several tissues and showed that it was produced locally independent of systemic RAS. The first demonstration of tissue Ang-II was in the arterial wall in sheep in 1980 [58]. Studies quantifying tissue Ang-II synthesis, using radiolabeled angiotensin, revealed that Ang-II in the heart, kidney, and adrenal gland [59,60] almost completely originates from local synthesis, both under normal and pathological conditions [60,61]. ACE was shown to be expressed in multiple tissues, including vascular endothelium, renal proximal tubular endothelium, heart, lung, small intestine, colon, activated macrophages, and several regions of the brain [62], where physiologic effects of ACE are the result of tissue rather than circulating ACE activity [63].

ACE is generally considered the main Ang-II-forming enzyme in the circulation. However, in tissues, various serine proteases were shown to play a role in Ang-II generation [53]. Not only chymase, but also trypsin [64] and kallikrein [65] serine proteases were shown to generate Ang-II in vitro and in vivo in ischemic dog hearts, ischemic human hearts, and even in normal healthy individuals during exercise [66]. In fact, chymase has been a focus of interest because of its specificity and potency in the human cardiovascular system [55,67].

Ang-II may exert local paracrine or autocrine effects through its locally expressed AT1 and AT2 receptors (Figure 1 and Table 1). AT1R was found to be expressed in several adult tissues, including blood vessels, heart, kidney, adrenal glands, and liver [2]. On the other hand, AT2R is mainly expressed in fetal tissue and decreases through fetal development [2] to be restricted to certain tissues, mainly the heart, vessels, brainstem, liver, and kidney [68]. At the tissue level, AT1R and AT2R exert opposite effects; therefore, the final local effects of Ang-II are defined by the combined net result obtained from the activation of both receptors. For instance, AT1R induces vasoconstriction and sodium retention in the kidney whereas AT2R promotes vasodilation and natriuresis [69]. On the other hand, in the gastrointestinal tract, AT2R opposes the actions of AT1R in sodium and water absorption, which contributes to the regulation of the finely tuned sodium transport in this tissue [70]. In general, AT2R stimulates protein dephosphorylation, which counterbalances protein phosphorylation induced by AT1R, thus, affecting the signaling pathways inside the cell, leading mainly to opposite cellular actions [69]. Despite this general "antagonistic" view of AT2R, certain studies on cardiac myocytes showed that its overexpression may complement, rather than antagonize, the AT1R effects in cellular hypertrophy [71,72]. Similarly, AT1R and AT2R synergistically act to induce adipogenesis and lipid storage in adipose tissue, wherein AT1R inhibit lipolysis, while AT2R induces the expression of lipogenic enzymes [73]. Interestingly, this adds a new level of complexity to RAS in which the effects of the system depend not only on the "inter-molecular" balance between the antagonistic arms, but also on the "intra-molecular" balance of the levels of the same molecule in certain cells under specific conditions.

Ang-II is the most studied pathway in RAS and additional research on it would open new avenues in understanding the complexity of the system and inter-pathway interactions.

3.4. Angiotensin-(1–7)

Ang-(1–7) was first discovered in rat brains in 1983 by Tonnaer and his colleagues [74]. However, at that time, it was thought to be an inactive peptide. The importance of Ang-(1–7) emerged in 1988 when it was found to be the major Ang-I-derived peptide in the presence and absence of ACE inhibition [75]. Ang-(1–7) was initially thought to exert its hypotensive effects in a bradykinin-dependent manner [76]. However, it was later demonstrated that Ang-(1–7) opposes the vasoconstrictive and proliferative actions of AT1R-mediated Ang-II actions [2,17]. In fact, the discovery of Ang-(1–7) and its effects lead to the belief that RAS local actions are mainly driven by the balance between the vasoconstrictor/proliferative and vasodilator/anti-proliferative actions of Ang-II and Ang-(1–7), respectivley [2].

Ang-(1–7) can be formed by different enzymes and pathways (Figure 1 and Table 1). The most potent and well known Ang-(1–7)-generating enzyme is ACE2 (angiotensin-I converting enzyme 2), which can generate Ang-(1–7) directly from Ang-II, or indirectly from Ang-I through Ang-(1–9) intermediate [77,78]. In fact, the former pathway is more favorable because the affinity of ACE2 to Ang-II is 400-folds greater than that to Ang-I [79]. Ang-(1–9) can be generated from Ang-I by the action of ACE2, cathepsin A (CTSA) [80], or carboxypeptidase A3 (CPA3), and then cleaved to form Ang-(1–7) by ACE [77], ACE2, or neprilysin (MME) (Figure 1 and Table 1). Alternatively, Ang-(1–7) can also be formed directly from Ang-I by prolylendopeptidase (PREP), thimet Oligopeptidase 1 (THOP1), [81] and Neurolysin (NLN) or from Ang-II cleavage by ACE2, PREP, and prolylcarboxipeptidase (PRCP) [2,79] (Figure 1 and Table 1).

In fact, ACE2 levels and the ACE/ACE2 ratio is generally considered a reference for Ang-(1–7) production. However, ACE2 is restricted to certain tissues and cells such as endothelial cells of the heart, kidneys, and testes [82]. In addition, the contribution of alternative enzymes in the production of Ang-(1–7) should be considered. For instance, metallopeptidase activity accounts for almost all Ang (1–7) production in atrial homogenate preparations, whereas Ang-II was produced equally by ACE and chymase while cathepsin A was responsible for 65% of the liberated Ang (1–9) [80]. This indicates that local angiotensin peptides production depends as well on the activity of "alternative" enzymes at the tissue level.

Ang-(1–7) exerts its effects mainly through the Mas receptor (MasR) (Figure 1 and Table 1). MasR was first described as Ang-(1–7) receptor in 2003, where its deletion abolished the binding of Ang-(1–7) to mouse kidneys, accompanied with the loss of Ang-(1–7)-induced relaxation [83]. By binding to MasR, Ang-(1–7) may induce many effects, antagonizing those of Ang-II/AT1R, such as vasodilation, inhibition of cell growth, anti-thrombosis, and anti-arrhythmogenic effects [84].

In addition, it was shown that MasR may antagonize AT1R in vitro and in vivo by forming a hetero-dimer with the AT1R, thus blocking the latter's activity [85]. Moreover, Ang-(1–7) can act on the AT2R (Figure 1 and Table 1), which exerts very similar effects to those induced by MasR [86]. In addition, emerging evidences raised controversies on the specificity of MasR to Ang-(1–7). Recently, MasR was shown to be stimulated by multiple other molecules such as Neuropeptide FF, Alamandine, Angiotensin III, Angiotensin IV, and Angioprotectin. Similarly, independent studies demonstrated the absence of MAS1 activation after Ang-(1–7) treatment in human mammary arteries from patients undergoing coronary revascularization surgery, splanchnic vessels from cirrhotic liver of human and rats and aorta from Sprague–Dawley rats [87].

Ang-(1–7) is present in the circulation, in addition to several other tissues and organs including the heart, blood vessels, kidney and liver [88], where it exerts local paracrine and autocrine actions. The alteration in circulatory and tissue Ang-(1–7) levels were shown to be associated with several diseases, including hypertension preeclampsia, hypertrophic myocardial disease, cognitive heart disease, myocardial infarction (MI), chronic kidney disease (CKD), and hepatic cirrhosis [2]. For instance, $ACE2^{-/-}$ mice developed age-dependent cardiomyopathy with increased oxidative stress, neutrophilic infiltration, inflammatory cytokine, and collagenase levels, mitogen-activated protein kinase (MAPK) activation and pathological hypertrophy [89]. These effects were inhibited by irbesartan, an AT1R blocker (ARB), which indicates a critical role for ACE2 in the suppression of Ang-II-mediated heart failure. In addition, a recent study suggested an important role for the ACE/ACE2 imbalance in the pathogenesis of severe acute pancreatitis where the ratio of pancreatic ACE2 to ACE expression was significantly reduced and paralleled the severity of the disease [90]. In another study, a reduction in ACE/ACE2 ratio was shown to be associated with acute respiratory distress syndrome, which was prevented by Ang-(1–7) or ARB treatment [91]. Recent studies have supported a metabolic role for the Ang-(1–7)/MasR arm in the liver and its counter-regulatory action to Ang-II/AT1R that interferes in several steps of intracellular insulin signaling arm in the pathophysiology of liver diseases [92]. Indeed, Ang-(1–7) has been shown to ameliorate glucose tolerance and to enhance insulin sensitivity, while Mas receptor has been described as an essential component of the insulin receptor signaling pathway [93]. Of interest, ACE2 treatment has been shown to ameliorate liver fibrosis through reduction of hepatic Ang-II levels concomitant with increased concentrations of Ang-(1–7) in liver tissue [94–96]. Moreover, Ang-(1–7)/MasR axis agonists may also play a role in the treatment of CKD by controlling the inflammatory response and fibrosis in kidney tissue [97].

Of note, high concentrations of Ang-(1–7) exerts biphasic effects on Na^+-, K^+-ATPase activity in a dose dependent manner by inducing similar effects to those induced by Ang-II at high concentrations, independent of MasR and AT2R, probably through the AT1R [98]. However, in the presence of Ang-II, Ang-(1–7) antagonized the stimulatory effects of Ang-II on Na^+, K^+-ATPase activity through a A779-sensitive receptor [99]. On the other hand, Ang-(1–7) infusion or MasR deficiency enhanced renal damage in models of renal insufficiency by aggravating the inflammatory response through NF-κB [100]. In contrast, another study showed that Ang-(1–7) suppressed inflammation by inhibiting the NF-κB pathway in rats with permanent cerebral ischaemia [101].

Taken together, these studies suggest that Ang-(1–7) exerts cell-specific effects based on its concentrations, available receptors, angiotensin peptides, and the physiological state of the tissue.

3.5. Angiotensin-III/-IV

Arterial concentration of Ang-III (hexapeptide 2–8) was first documented in 1980 in sheep, and accounted for 42% of that of Ang-II [58]. Ang-III is generated from Ang-II by the removal of the first amino terminus aa by Aminopeptidase A (ENPEP) [8] (Figure 1 and Table 1). In addition, it can be generated from Ang-I by a two-steps pathway involving ENPEP and ACE, respectively [102]. Studies have shown that Ang-III exerts similar, but less potent, actions as compared to Ang-II [2,103], by acting on AT1R and AT2R, with higher affinity to the former [104]. Indeed, Ang-III was shown to increase blood pressure, vasopressin and aldosterone release, in addition to inducing inflammatory genes expression [2,103].

Ang-III in turn can be converted into Ang-IV (pentapeptide 3–8) by the action of the aminopeptidase N (ANPEP) [105], and possibly aminopeptidase B (RNPEP) [106] (Figure 1 and Table 1). Ang-IV acts through its Angiotensin type 4 receptor (AT4R), which is the insulin-regulated membrane aminopeptidase (IRAP). The latter is a type II integral membrane spanning protein belonging to the M1 family of aminopeptidases that is expressed in several tissues, including the brain, adrenal gland, kidney, lung, liver, and heart [107] (Figure 1 and Table 1).

Recent studies have shown that certain local Ang-II-mediated effects could be attributed to Ang-III. For example, Padia et al. showed that the conversion of Ang-II to Ang-III is critical for AT2R-mediated natriuresis in Sprague–Dawley rats [104]. Similarly, in Wistar rats, the Ang-II-mediated enhancement in baroreceptor heart reflex was abrogated in the presence of ENPEP inhibitor, indicating that Ang-III is the active angiotensin peptide involved in central blood pressure regulation [108]. On the other hand, Handa et al. showed that intrarenal injection of Ang I, Ang-II, or Ang-III induce dose-dependent vasoconstriction in Sprague–Dawley rats. However, Ang-IV or Ang-(3–10) injection produced a dose-dependent rapid vasoconstriction, lasting for seconds, followed by a transient vasodilatation, lasting for minutes [109]. This indicates that RAS induces peptide-specific effects at the tissue level.

The major effects of AT4R activation are thought to be in the brain where it can enhance learning and memory [107]. However, the mechanism by which Ang-IV exerts its effects through IRAP is still not clear [110]. One suggestion is that Ang-IV inhibits the catalytic activity of IRAP, thereby extending the half-life of its neuropeptide substrates. Another suggestion is that it may modulate glucose uptake by modulating GLUT4 trafficking. Others suggest that it may act directly on cellular mechanisms by inducing cellular signaling after its binding [110]. Ang-IV in the brain was also shown to be implicated in regulating blood pressure by acting on the AT1R [111], which was shown to mediate several Ang-IV effects. Indeed, Ang-IV mediates pressure and renal vasoconstrictor effects in mice via AT1a receptor whereas AT4R is not involved [112]. Finally, Ang-IV-mediated non-prostaglandin renal vasodilatory activity was found to be linked to renal vascular AT1R [109].

The Ang-III/Ang-IV axes have added a new level of complexity to the system and identified novel mechanisms by which Ang-II may exert its effects. This needs to be further studied to elucidate possible flows in the interpretation of the effects of Ang-II agonists and to identify possible mechanisms that would improve Ang-II antagonists' mode of action.

3.6. Angiotensin A/Alamandine/MrgD

Ang-A is a recently discovered angiotensin peptide detected in the plasma of patients with end-stage renal disease, where Ang-A/Ang-II ratio was found to be higher compared to healthy individuals [113]. Ang-A is an octapeptide with the sequence Ala-Arg-Val-Tyr-Ile-His-Pro-Phe, which can be produced from Ang-II by conversion of the first amino acid, aspartic acid, into alanine [113]. Ang-A can bind to AT1R and AT2R with equal affinity as Ang-II [114]. Intravenous and intrarenal administration of Ang A induced dose-dependent increase in blood pressure and renal vasoconstrictor responses in normotensive and spontaneously hypertensive rats [114,115]. In isolated perfused rat kidney, Ang-A induced smaller vasoconstrictive effects compared to Ang-II, which were inhibited using AT1R inhibitor, but not AT2R inhibitor [113,114].

In fact, the importance of Ang-A is increasing due to its junctional position in the system. Despite its vasoconstrictive and pro-proliferative actions, Ang-A is also a precursor of alamandine, a recently discovered peptide identified in rats, mice, and humans [116]. Alamandine can also be produced from Ang-(1–7) by ACE2 and was shown to produce several physiological actions that resemble those produced by Ang-(1–7) including vasodilation, antifibrotic, antihypertensive, and CNS effects, independent of MasR and AT2R [116]. The effects of alamandine were shown to be mediated through the activation of a specific receptor, the member D of Mas1-related G-protein-coupled receptor (MasDR) [116], which has been recently demonstrated to also be an alternative receptor to

Ang-(1–7) [117]. Interestingly, alamandine was shown to exert opposite effects in central nervous system where microinjection of alamandine into the rostral ventrolateral medulla of rats induced a vasopressor effect, whereas its administration into the caudal ventrolateral medulla elicited a vasodilatory effect. Of importance, similar effects were obtained after Ang-(1–7) injection [116]. On the other hand, in control but not diseased blood vessels, alamandine enhanced acetylcholine-mediated vasodilation in normal thoracic aorta and the iliac artery, whereas it reduced it in the renal artery [118]. Interestingly, these effects were absent in blood vessels from atherogenic rabbits, which also showed a reduced vasoconstrictive response toward Ang-A.

The finding of MasDR receptor has added another level of complexity into RAS, especially with regards to the anti-inflammatory Ang-(1–7) axis. This warrants further studies that may explain additional interactions and would balance between the different axes of RAS.

3.7. Other Angiotensin Peptides

Ang-(1–9) was considered for a long time as an intermediate peptide with no biological significance. However, recent evidence suggests that Ang-(1–9) can exert several effects in vivo and in vitro independent of Ang-(1–7)-mediated MasR activation, possibly through AT2R [2]. Indeed, a new study showed that Ang-(1–9) exerts beneficial cardiovascular effects via the AT2R in hypertensive rats independent of blood pressure modulation, where it ameliorated structural alterations (hypertrophy and fibrosis) and oxidative stress in the heart and aorta and improved cardiac and endothelial function [2]. These effects were inhibited by an AT2R antagonist, but not a MasR one. On the contrary, in another study on rats, Ang-(1–9) enhanced thrombosis, decreased plasma concentrations of tissue plasminogen activator (tPA), and increased the levels of its inhibitor (PAI-1) through indirect activation of AT1R [119]. These effects were reversed by selective antagonists to AT1R, but not to that of Ang-(1–7).

Ang-(3–7) is an angiotensin peptide that was shown to bind to AT4R, with lower affinity compared to Ang-IV, leading to important effects in the brain and kidney [2]. Ang-(3–7) can be produced by cleavage of Ang-(1–7), Ang-II, or Ang-IV by aminopeptidases or carboxypeptidases [2]. Administration of Ang (3–7) intracerebroventricularly (i. c. v.) significantly enhanced learning and behavioral activity in rats [120]. Co-treatment withthe ARB, losartan, only affected learning ability, without altering the behavioral activity. This suggests that Ang (3–7) is an active peptide that exerts its effects through different receptors, one of which is AT1R [120]. Moreover, Ang-(1–7) induced inhibitory effects on the energy-dependent solute transport in proximal tubules of the rat kidney [121] were shown to be mediated by the metabolism of Ang-(1–7) into Ang (3–7), by binding to AT4R [121]. Such results may raise questions about the previously described "direct" effects of certain angiotensin peptides.

4. Conclusion and Future Directions

The concept of tissue RAS could be defined as a specific combination of RAS enzymes that are locally expressed in a tissue, which results in the production of a specific quantitative and qualitative combination of peptides that can bind to their corresponding locally expressed receptors, thus leading to a locally balanced paracrine/autocrine effect that plays a role in tissue physiology and homeostasis. A change in local RAS expression will consequently lead to alterations in the balance obtained, and thus, to pathophysiological consequences (Figure 2). In this regard, studies on RAS need to be shifted from the one peptide-one pathway approach, toward a more general approach that considers the tissue-specific pathways and their respective local and systemic interactions. Indeed, the knowledge obtained from the former approach may lead to misleading conclusions that rely on the used model, with a lack of information on other pathways that may balance the effect of the pathway in question. Therefore, for a better understanding of the "real" global physiological effects of RAS, it is necessary to measure the different components of RAS in a specific tissue, under specific physiological conditions.

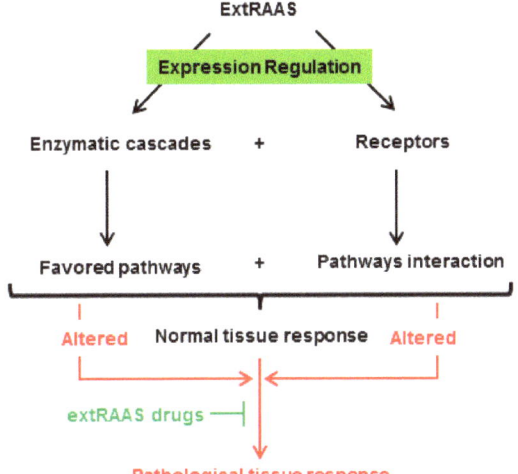

Figure 2. A specific combination of locally expressed RAS enzymes in a tissue results in the production of a specific combination of peptides that can bind to their corresponding receptors, leading to a locally balanced paracrine/autocrine effect that plays a role in tissue physiology and homeostasis. A change in local balance of RAS components will consequently lead to pathophysiological consequences.

Using transcriptomics meta-analysis, we have recently established the atlas of tissue RAS, which includes the transcriptional maps of RAS in 23 normal human tissues [7,122]. The maps provide information on the favored pathways of RAS in each tissue, but also on the co-expression of RAS genes, which may provide the basis for the discovery of potential regulatory mechanisms involved in the global expression of RAS components at the tissue level. In this regard, we have recently created the transcriptional maps of RAS in normal and atherosclerotic vascular wall showing the differences in angiotensin metabolism between both tissues [123]. Also, by analyzing the promoters of co-expressed genes, we identified potential transcription factors that could play a role in the global expression of RAS components in atheroma. Therefore, the atlas needs to be extended and studied at the protein level. In addition, RAS maps should be established from studies on each tissue under pathophysiological conditions, which will help understand the way the system is altered in each tissue under specific conditions, and thus, a better understanding of the mechanisms by which the system is involved in local tissue pathophysiology.

Funding: This work was supported by grants to KZ from Coopération pour l'Évaluation et le Développement de la Recherche (CEDRE), the Lebanese National Council for Scientific Research (CNRS) and Lebanese University grants. A.N. was awarded a scholarship from "La Nouvelle Société Francophone d'Athérosclérose" (NSFA).

Conflicts of Interest: The authors declare no conflict of interest.

References

1. Bader, M. Tissue renin-angiotensin-aldosterone systems: Targets for pharmacological therapy. *Annu. Rev. Pharmacol. Toxicol.* **2010**, *50*, 439–465. [CrossRef] [PubMed]
2. Ribeiro-Oliveira, A.; Nogueira, A.I.; Pereira, R.M.; Boas, W.W.V.; dos Santos, R.A.S.; e Silva, A.C.S. The renin–angiotensin system and diabetes: An update. *Vasc. Health Risk Manag.* **2008**, *4*, 787–803. [PubMed]
3. Nehme, A.; Zibara, K. Cellular distribution and interaction between extended renin-angiotensin-aldosterone system pathways in atheroma. *Atherosclerosis* **2017**, *263*, 334–342. [CrossRef]
4. Nehme, A.; Zibara, K. Efficiency and specificity of RAAS inhibitors in cardiovascular diseases: How to achieve better end-organ protection? *Hypertens. Res.* **2017**, *40*, 903–909. [CrossRef] [PubMed]

5. Borghi, C.; SIIA Task Force; Rossi, F.; SIF Task Force. Role of the Renin-Angiotensin-Aldosterone System and Its Pharmacological Inhibitors in Cardiovascular Diseases: Complex and Critical Issues. *High Blood Press Cardiovasc. Prev.* **2015**, *22*, 429–444. [CrossRef] [PubMed]

6. Deschepper, C.F. Angiotensinogen: Hormonal regulation and relative importance in the generation of angiotensin II. *Kidney Int.* **1994**, *46*, 1561–1563. [CrossRef] [PubMed]

7. Nehme, A.; Cerutti, C.; Dhaouadi, N.; Gustin, M.P.; Courand, P.-Y.; Zibara, K.; Bricca, G. Atlas of tissue renin-angiotensin-aldosterone system in human: A transcriptomic meta-analysis. *Sci Rep* **2015**, *5*, 10035. [CrossRef]

8. Atlas, S.A. The renin-angiotensin aldosterone system: Pathophysiological role and pharmacologic inhibition. *J. Manag. Care Pharm.* **2007**, *13*, 9–20. [CrossRef] [PubMed]

9. Dzau, V.J.; Herrmann, H.C. Hormonal control of angiotensinogen production. *Life Sci.* **1982**, *30*, 577–584. [CrossRef]

10. Hsueh, W.A. Potential effects of renin activation on the regulation of renin production. *Am. J. Physiol.* **1984**, *247*, F205–F212. [CrossRef]

11. Kohlstedt, K.; Busse, R.; Fleming, I. Signaling via the angiotensin-converting enzyme enhances the expression of cyclooxygenase-2 in endothelial cells. *Hypertension* **2005**, *45*, 126–132. [CrossRef] [PubMed]

12. Gasparo, M.; de Catt, K.J.; Inagami, T.; Wright, J.W.; Unger, T. International Union of Pharmacology. XXIII. The Angiotensin II Receptors. *Pharmacol. Rev.* **2000**, *52*, 415–472.

13. Kim, S.; Iwao, H. Molecular and Cellular Mechanisms of Angiotensin II-Mediated Cardiovascular and Renal Diseases. *Pharmacol. Rev.* **2000**, *52*, 11–34. [PubMed]

14. Jaffe, I.Z.; Mendelsohn, M.E. Angiotensin II and aldosterone regulate gene transcription via functional mineralocortocoid receptors in human coronary artery smooth muscle cells. *Circ. Res.* **2005**, *96*, 643–650. [CrossRef] [PubMed]

15. Bhargava, A.; Wang, J.; Pearce, D. Regulation of epithelial ion transport by aldosterone through changes in gene expression. *Mol. Cell. Endocrinol.* **2004**, *217*, 189–196. [CrossRef]

16. Verhovez, A.; Williams, T.A.; Morello, F.; Monticone, S.; Brizzi, M.F.; Dentelli, P.; Fallo, F.; Fabris, B.; Amenta, F.; Gomez-Sanchez, C.; et al. Aldosterone does not modify gene expression in human endothelial cells. *Horm. Metab. Res.* **2012**, *44*, 234–238. [CrossRef] [PubMed]

17. Ferrario, C.M.; Ahmad, S.; Nagata, S.; Simington, S.W.; Varagic, J.; Kon, N.; Dell'italia, L.J. An evolving story of angiotensin-II-forming pathways in rodents and humans. *Clin. Sci.* **2014**, *126*, 461–469. [CrossRef]

18. Ganten, D.; Minnich, J.L.; Granger, P.; Hayduk, K.; Brecht, H.M.; Barbeau, A.; Boucher, R.; Genest, J. Angiotensin-forming enzyme in brain tissue. *Science* **1971**, *173*, 64–65. [CrossRef] [PubMed]

19. Husain, A.; Bumpus, F.M.; Smeby, R.R.; Brosnihan, K.B.; Khosla, M.C.; Speth, R.C.; Ferrario, C.M. Evidence for the existence of a family of biologically active angiotensin I-like peptides in the dog central nervous system. *Circ. Res.* **1983**, *52*, 460–464. [CrossRef] [PubMed]

20. Nguyen, G.; Delarue, F.; Burcklé, C.; Bouzhir, L.; Giller, T.; Sraer, J.-D. Pivotal role of the renin/prorenin receptor in angiotensin II production and cellular responses to renin. *J. Clin. Invest.* **2002**, *109*, 1417–1427. [CrossRef]

21. Paul, M.; Mehr, A.P.; Kreutz, R. Physiology of Local Renin-Angiotensin Systems. *Physiol. Rev.* **2006**, *86*, 747–803. [CrossRef] [PubMed]

22. Lau, T.; Carlsson, P.-O.; Leung, P.S. Evidence for a local angiotensin-generating system and dose-dependent inhibition of glucose-stimulated insulin release by angiotensin II in isolated pancreatic islets. *Diabetologia* **2004**, *47*, 240–248. [CrossRef] [PubMed]

23. Dzau, V.J. Circulating versus local renin-angiotensin system in cardiovascular homeostasis. *Circulation* **1988**, *77*, I4–I13. [PubMed]

24. Dzau, V.J. Tissue renin-angiotensin system in myocardial hypertrophy and failure. *Arch. Intern. Med.* **1993**, *153*, 937–942. [CrossRef] [PubMed]

25. Wu, C.; Lu, H.; Cassis, L.A.; Daugherty, A. Molecular and Pathophysiological Features of Angiotensinogen: A Mini Review. *N. Am. J. Med. Sci. (Boston)* **2011**, *4*, 183–190. [CrossRef]

26. Batenburg, W.W.; Danser, A.H.J. (Pro)renin and its receptors: Pathophysiological implications. *Clin. Sci.* **2012**, *123*, 121–133. [CrossRef] [PubMed]

27. Kaneshiro, Y.; Ichihara, A.; Sakoda, M.; Takemitsu, T.; Nabi, A.H.M.N.; Uddin, M.N.; Nakagawa, T.; Nishiyama, A.; Suzuki, F.; Inagami, T.; et al. Slowly progressive, angiotensin II-independent

glomerulosclerosis in human (pro)renin receptor-transgenic rats. *J. Am. Soc. Nephrol.* **2007**, *18*, 1789–1795. [CrossRef] [PubMed]

28. Lutterotti, N.; von Catanzaro, D.F.; Sealey, J.E.; Laragh, J.H. Renin is not synthesized by cardiac and extrarenal vascular tissues. A review of experimental evidence. *Circulation* **1994**, *89*, 458–470. [CrossRef]

29. Boddi, M.; Poggesi, L.; Coppo, M.; Zarone, N.; Sacchi, S.; Tania, C.; Neri Serneri, G.G. Human vascular renin-angiotensin system and its functional changes in relation to different sodium intakes. *Hypertension* **1998**, *31*, 836–842. [CrossRef]

30. Neri Serneri, G.G.; Boddi, M.; Coppo, M.; Chechi, T.; Zarone, N.; Moira, M.; Poggesi, L.; Margheri, M.; Simonetti, I. Evidence for the existence of a functional cardiac renin-angiotensin system in humans. *Circulation* **1996**, *94*, 1886–1893. [CrossRef]

31. Cassis, L.A.; Police, S.B.; Yiannikouris, F.; Thatcher, S.E. Local adipose tissue renin-angiotensin system. *Curr. Hypertens. Rep.* **2008**, *10*, 93–98. [CrossRef]

32. Santos, C.F.; Akashi, A.E.; Dionísio, T.J.; Sipert, C.R.; Didier, D.N.; Greene, A.S.; Oliveira, S.H.P.; Pereira, H.J.V.; Becari, C.; Oliveira, E.B.; et al. Characterization of a local renin-angiotensin system in rat gingival tissue. *J. Periodontol.* **2009**, *80*, 130–139. [CrossRef] [PubMed]

33. Saris, J.J.; Derkx, F.H.; De Bruin, R.J.; Dekkers, D.H.; Lamers, J.M.; Saxena, P.R.; Schalekamp, M.A.; Jan Danser, A.H. High-affinity prorenin binding to cardiac man-6-P/IGF-II receptors precedes proteolytic activation to renin. *Am. J. Physiol. Heart Circ. Physiol.* **2001**, *280*, H1706–H1715. [CrossRef] [PubMed]

34. Morris, B.J.; Reid, I.A. A "Renin-Like" Enzymatic Action of Cathepsin D and the Similarity in Subcellular Distributions of "Renin-Like" Activity and Cathepsin D in the Midbrain of Dogs. *Endocrinology* **1978**, *103*, 1289–1296. [CrossRef] [PubMed]

35. Rakoczy, P.E.; Sarks, S.H.; Daw, N.; Constable, I.J. Distribution of cathepsin D in human eyes with or without age-related maculopathy. *Exp. Eye Res.* **1999**, *69*, 367–374. [CrossRef] [PubMed]

36. Naseem, R.H.; Hedegard, W.; Henry, T.D.; Lessard, J.; Sutter, K.; Katz, S.A. Plasma cathepsin D isoforms and their active metabolites increase after myocardial infarction and contribute to plasma renin activity. *Basic Res. Cardiol.* **2005**, *100*, 139–146. [CrossRef] [PubMed]

37. Lavrentyev, E.N.; Estes, A.M.; Malik, K.U. Mechanism of high glucose induced angiotensin II production in rat vascular smooth muscle cells. *Circ. Res.* **2007**, *101*, 455–464. [CrossRef] [PubMed]

38. Belova, L.A. Angiotensin II-generating enzymes. *Biochemistry Mosc.* **2000**, *65*, 1337–1345. [CrossRef] [PubMed]

39. Hackenthal, E.; Hackenthal, R.; Hilgenfeldt, U. Isorenin, pseudorenin, cathepsin D and renin. A comparative enzymatic study of angiotensin-forming enzymes. *Biochim. Biophys. Acta* **1978**, *522*, 574–588. [CrossRef]

40. Figueiredo, A.F.; Takii, Y.; Tsuji, H.; Kato, K.; Inagami, T. Rat kidney renin and cathepsin D: Purification and comparison of properties. *Biochemistry* **1983**, *22*, 5476–5481. [CrossRef]

41. Nagata, S.; Kato, J.; Sasaki, K.; Minamino, N.; Eto, T.; Kitamura, K. Isolation and identification of proangiotensin-12, a possible component of the renin-angiotensin system. *Biochem. Biophys. Res. Commun.* **2006**, *350*, 1026–1031. [CrossRef] [PubMed]

42. Komatsu, Y.; Kida, N.; Nozaki, N.; Kuwasako, K.; Nagata, S.; Kitamura, K.; Kato, J. Effects of proangiotensin-12 infused continuously over 14 days in conscious rats. *Eur. J. Pharmacol.* **2012**, *683*, 186–189. [CrossRef]

43. Ferrario, C.M.; Von Cannon, J.; Jiao, Y.; Ahmad, S.; Bader, M.; Dell'Italia, L.J.; Groban, L.; Varagic, J. Cardiac angiotensin-(1–12) expression and systemic hypertension in rats expressing the human angiotensinogen gene. *Am. J. Physiol. Heart Circ. Physiol.* **2016**, *310*, H995–H1002. [CrossRef] [PubMed]

44. Isa, K.; García-Espinosa, M.A.; Arnold, A.C.; Pirro, N.T.; Tommasi, E.N.; Ganten, D.; Chappell, M.C.; Ferrario, C.M.; Diz, D.I. Chronic immunoneutralization of brain angiotensin-(1–12) lowers blood pressure in transgenic (mRen2)27 hypertensive rats. *Am. J. Physiol. Regul. Integr. Comp. Physiol.* **2009**, *297*, R111–R115. [CrossRef]

45. Arnold, A.C.; Isa, K.; Shaltout, H.A.; Nautiyal, M.; Ferrario, C.M.; Chappell, M.C.; Diz, D.I. Angiotensin-(1–12) requires angiotensin converting enzyme and AT1 receptors for cardiovascular actions within the solitary tract nucleus. *Am. J. Physiol. Heart Circ. Physiol.* **2010**, *299*, H763–H771. [CrossRef]

46. Chitravanshi, V.C.; Sapru, H.N. Cardiovascular responses elicited by a new endogenous angiotensin in the nucleus tractus solitarius of the rat. *Am. J. Physiol. Heart Circ. Physiol.* **2011**, *300*, H230–H240. [CrossRef] [PubMed]

47. Chitravanshi, V.C.; Proddutur, A.; Sapru, H.N. Cardiovascular actions of angiotensin-(1–12) in the hypothalamic paraventricular nucleus of the rat are mediated via angiotensin II. *Exp. Physiol.* **2012**, *97*, 1001–1017. [CrossRef]

48. Jessup, J.A.; Trask, A.J.; Chappell, M.C.; Nagata, S.; Kato, J.; Kitamura, K.; Ferrario, C.M. Localization of the novel angiotensin peptide, angiotensin-(1–12), in heart and kidney of hypertensive and normotensive rats. *Am. J. Physiol. Heart Circ. Physiol.* **2008**, *294*, H2614–H2618. [CrossRef]

49. Nagata, S.; Kato, J.; Kuwasako, K.; Kitamura, K. Plasma and tissue levels of proangiotensin-12 and components of the renin-angiotensin system (RAS) following low- or high-salt feeding in rats. *Peptides* **2010**, *31*, 889–892. [CrossRef] [PubMed]

50. Westwood, B.M.; Chappell, M.C. Divergent pathways for the angiotensin-(1–12) metabolism in the rat circulation and kidney. *Peptides* **2012**, *35*, 190–195. [CrossRef] [PubMed]

51. Ahmad, S.; Varagic, J.; Westwood, B.M.; Chappell, M.C.; Ferrario, C.M. Uptake and metabolism of the novel peptide angiotensin-(1–12) by neonatal cardiac myocytes. *PLoS ONE* **2011**, *6*, e15759. [CrossRef]

52. Ahmad, S.; Simmons, T.; Varagic, J.; Moniwa, N.; Chappell, M.C.; Ferrario, C.M. Chymase-dependent generation of angiotensin II from angiotensin-(1–12) in human atrial tissue. *PLoS ONE* **2011**, *6*, e28501. [CrossRef]

53. Prosser, H.C.; Richards, A.M.; Forster, M.E.; Pemberton, C.J. Regional vascular response to ProAngiotensin-12 (PA12) through the rat arterial system. *Peptides* **2010**, *31*, 1540–1545. [CrossRef] [PubMed]

54. Tonnesen, M.G.; Klempner, M.S.; Austen, K.F.; Wintroub, B.U. Identification of a human neutrophil angiotension II-generating protease as cathepsin G. *J. Clin. Invest.* **1982**, *69*, 25–30. [CrossRef]

55. Urata, H.; Kinoshita, A.; Misono, K.S.; Bumpus, F.M.; Husain, A. Identification of a highly specific chymase as the major angiotensin II-forming enzyme in the human heart. *J. Biol. Chem.* **1990**, *265*, 22348–22357. [PubMed]

56. Park, S.; Bivona, B.J.; Kobori, H.; Seth, D.M.; Chappell, M.C.; Lazartigues, E.; Harrison-Bernard, L.M. Major role for ACE-independent intrarenal ANG II formation in type II diabetes. *Am. J. Physiol. Renal Physiol.* **2010**, *298*, F37–F48. [CrossRef] [PubMed]

57. Nouet, S.; Nahmias, C. Signal transduction from the angiotensin II AT2 receptor. *Trends Endocrinol. Metab.* **2000**, *11*, 1–6. [CrossRef]

58. Fei, D.T.; Coghlan, J.P.; Fernley, R.T.; Scoggins, B.A.; Tregear, G.W. Peripheral production of angiotensin II and III in sheep. *Circ. Res.* **1980**, *46*, I135–I137.

59. Van Kats, J.P.; van Meegen, J.R.; Verdouw, P.D.; Duncker, D.J.; Schalekamp, M.A.; Danser, A.H. Subcellular localization of angiotensin II in kidney and adrenal. *J. Hypertens.* **2001**, *19*, 583–589. [CrossRef] [PubMed]

60. Van Kats, J.P.; Danser, A.H.; van Meegen, J.R.; Sassen, L.M.; Verdouw, P.D.; Schalekamp, M.A. Angiotensin production by the heart: A quantitative study in pigs with the use of radiolabeled angiotensin infusions. *Circulation* **1998**, *98*, 73–81. [CrossRef]

61. Danser, A.H.; van Kats, J.P.; Verdouw, P.D.; Schalekamp, M.A. Evidence for the existence of a functional cardiac renin-angiotensin system in humans. *Circulation* **1997**, *96*, 3795–3796. [PubMed]

62. Sealey, J.E. Evidence for cardiovascular effects of prorenin. *J. Hum. Hypertens.* **1995**, *9*, 381–384.

63. Esther, C.R.; Marino, E.M.; Howard, T.E.; Machaud, A.; Corvol, P.; Capecchi, M.R.; Bernstein, K.E. The critical role of tissue angiotensin-converting enzyme as revealed by gene targeting in mice. *J. Clin. Invest.* **1997**, *99*, 2375–2385. [CrossRef]

64. Arakawa, K.; Ikeda, M.; Fukuyama, J.; Sakai, T. A pressor formation by trypsin from renin-denatured human plasma protein. *J. Clin. Endocrinol. Metab.* **1976**, *42*, 599–602. [CrossRef]

65. Arakawa, K.; Maruta, H. Ability of kallikrein to generate angiotensin II-like pressor substance and a proposed 'kinin-tensin enzyme system'. *Nature* **1980**, *288*, 705–706. [CrossRef] [PubMed]

66. Miura, S.; Ideishi, M.; Sakai, T.; Motoyama, M.; Kinoshita, A.; Sasaguri, M.; Tanaka, H.; Shindo, M.; Arakawa, K. Angiotensin II formation by an alternative pathway during exercise in humans. *J. Hypertens.* **1994**, *12*, 1177–1181. [CrossRef] [PubMed]

67. Arakawa, K.; Urata, H. Hypothesis regarding the pathophysiological role of alternative pathways of angiotensin II formation in atherosclerosis. *Hypertension* **2000**, *36*, 638–641. [CrossRef] [PubMed]

68. Li, Y.; Li, X.-H.; Yuan, H. Angiotensin II type-2 receptor-specific effects on the cardiovascular system. *Cardiovasc. Diagn. Ther.* **2012**, *2*, 56–62. [PubMed]

69. Carey, R.M.; Wang, Z.Q.; Siragy, H.M. Update: Role of the angiotensin type-2 (AT(2)) receptor in blood pressure regulation. *Curr. Hypertens. Rep.* **2000**, *2*, 198–201. [CrossRef] [PubMed]
70. Jin, X.H.; Wang, Z.Q.; Siragy, H.M.; Guerrant, R.L.; Carey, R.M. Regulation of jejunal sodium and water absorption by angiotensin subtype receptors. *Am. J. Physiol.* **1998**, *275*, R515–R523. [CrossRef]
71. Strauss, M.H.; Hall, A.S. Angiotensin Receptor Blockers May Increase Risk of Myocardial Infarction. *Circulation* **2006**, *114*, 838–854. [CrossRef]
72. Reudelhuber, T.L. The continuing saga of the AT2 receptor: A case of the good, the bad, and the innocuous. *Hypertension* **2005**, *46*, 1261–1262. [CrossRef]
73. Pahlavani, M.; Kalupahana, N.S.; Ramalingam, L.; Moustaid-Moussa, N. Regulation and Functions of the Renin-Angiotensin System in White and Brown Adipose Tissue. *Compr Physiol* **2017**, *7*, 1137–1150.
74. Tonnaer, J.A.; Engels, G.M.; Wiegant, V.M.; Burbach, J.P.; De Jong, W.; De Wied, D. Proteolytic conversion of angiotensins in rat brain tissue. *Eur. J. Biochem.* **1983**, *131*, 415–421. [CrossRef]
75. Santos, R.A.; Brosnihan, K.B.; Chappell, M.C.; Pesquero, J.; Chernicky, C.L.; Greene, L.J.; Ferrario, C.M. Converting enzyme activity and angiotensin metabolism in the dog brainstem. *Hypertension* **1988**, *11*, I153–I157. [CrossRef]
76. Tom, B.; Dendorfer, A.; Danser, A.H.J. Bradykinin, angiotensin-(1–7), and ACE inhibitors: How do they interact? *Int. J. Biochem. Cell Biol.* **2003**, *35*, 792–801. [CrossRef]
77. Donoghue, M.; Hsieh, F.; Baronas, E.; Godbout, K.; Gosselin, M.; Stagliano, N.; Donovan, M.; Woolf, B.; Robison, K.; Jeyaseelan, R.; et al. A novel angiotensin-converting enzyme-related carboxypeptidase (ACE2) converts angiotensin I to angiotensin 1–9. *Circ. Res.* **2000**, *87*, E1–E9. [CrossRef]
78. Tipnis, S.R.; Hooper, N.M.; Hyde, R.; Karran, E.; Christie, G.; Turner, A.J. A Human Homolog of Angiotensin-converting Enzyme CLONING AND FUNCTIONAL EXPRESSION AS A CAPTOPRIL-INSENSITIVE CARBOXYPEPTIDASE. *J. Biol. Chem.* **2000**, *275*, 33238–33243. [CrossRef]
79. Rice, G.I.; Thomas, D.A.; Grant, P.J.; Turner, A.J.; Hooper, N.M. Evaluation of angiotensin-converting enzyme (ACE), its homologue ACE2 and neprilysin in angiotensin peptide metabolism. *Biochem. J.* **2004**, *383*, 45–51. [CrossRef]
80. Jackman, H.L.; Massad, M.G.; Sekosan, M.; Tan, F.; Brovkovych, V.; Marcic, B.M.; Erdös, E.G. Angiotensin 1–9 and 1–7 release in human heart: Role of cathepsin A. *Hypertension* **2002**, *39*, 976–981. [CrossRef]
81. Pereira, M.G.A.G.; Souza, L.L.; Becari, C.; Duarte, D.A.; Camacho, F.R.B.; Oliveira, J.A.C.; Gomes, M.D.; Oliveira, E.B.; Salgado, M.C.O.; Garcia-Cairasco, N.; et al. Angiotensin II-independent angiotensin-(1–7) formation in rat hippocampus: Involvement of thimet oligopeptidase. *Hypertension* **2013**, *62*, 879–885. [CrossRef]
82. Douglas, G.C.; O'Bryan, M.K.; Hedger, M.P.; Lee, D.K.L.; Yarski, M.A.; Smith, A.I.; Lew, R.A. The novel angiotensin-converting enzyme (ACE) homolog, ACE2, is selectively expressed by adult Leydig cells of the testis. *Endocrinology* **2004**, *145*, 4703–4711. [CrossRef]
83. Santos, R.A.S.; Simoes e Silva, A.C.; Maric, C.; Silva, D.M.R.; Machado, R.P.; de Buhr, I.; Heringer-Walther, S.; Pinheiro, S.V.B.; Lopes, M.T.; Bader, M.; et al. Angiotensin-(1–7) is an endogenous ligand for the G protein-coupled receptor Mas. *Proc. Natl. Acad. Sci. USA* **2003**, *100*, 8258–8263. [CrossRef] [PubMed]
84. Simões e Silva, A.C.; Silveira, K.D.; Ferreira, A.J.; Teixeira, M.M. ACE2, angiotensin-(1–7) and Mas receptor axis in inflammation and fibrosis. *Br. J. Pharmacol.* **2013**, *169*, 477–492. [CrossRef] [PubMed]
85. Kostenis, E.; Milligan, G.; Christopoulos, A.; Sanchez-Ferrer, C.F.; Heringer-Walther, S.; Sexton, P.M.; Gembardt, F.; Kellett, E.; Martini, L.; Vanderheyden, P.; et al. G-protein-coupled receptor Mas is a physiological antagonist of the angiotensin II type 1 receptor. *Circulation* **2005**, *111*, 1806–1813. [CrossRef] [PubMed]
86. Villela, D.; Leonhardt, J.; Patel, N.; Joseph, J.; Kirsch, S.; Hallberg, A.; Unger, T.; Bader, M.; Santos, R.A.; Sumners, C.; et al. Angiotensin type 2 receptor (AT2R) and receptor Mas: A complex liaison. *Clin. Sci.* **2015**, *128*, 227–234. [CrossRef] [PubMed]
87. Karnik, S.S.; Khuraijam, D.; Tirupula, K.; Unal, H. Significance of Ang(1–7) coupling with MAS1 and other GPCRs to the Renin-Angiotensin System: IUPHAR Review "X". *Br. J. Pharmacol.* **2017**. [CrossRef]
88. Chappell, M.C. Emerging evidence for a functional angiotensin-converting enzyme 2-angiotensin-(1–7)-MAS receptor axis: More than regulation of blood pressure? *Hypertension* **2007**, *50*, 596–599. [CrossRef] [PubMed]

89. Oudit, G.Y.; Kassiri, Z.; Patel, M.P.; Chappell, M.; Butany, J.; Backx, P.H.; Tsushima, R.G.; Scholey, J.W.; Khokha, R.; Penninger, J.M. Angiotensin II-mediated oxidative stress and inflammation mediate the age-dependent cardiomyopathy in ACE2 null mice. *Cardiovasc. Res.* **2007**, *75*, 29–39. [CrossRef]

90. Liu, R.; Qi, H.; Wang, J.; Wang, Y.; Cui, L.; Wen, Y.; Yin, C. Angiotensin-converting enzyme (ACE and ACE2) imbalance correlates with the severity of cerulein-induced acute pancreatitis in mice. *Exp. Physiol.* **2014**, *99*, 651–663. [CrossRef]

91. Wösten-van Asperen, R.M.; Lutter, R.; Specht, P.A.; Moll, G.N.; van Woensel, J.B.; van der Loos, C.M.; van Goor, H.; Kamilic, J.; Florquin, S.; Bos, A.P. Acute respiratory distress syndrome leads to reduced ratio of ACE/ACE2 activities and is prevented by angiotensin-(1–7) or an angiotensin II receptor antagonist. *J. Pathol.* **2011**, *225*, 618–627. [CrossRef]

92. Simões e Silva, A.C.; Miranda, A.S.; Rocha, N.P.; Teixeira, A.L. Renin angiotensin system in liver diseases: Friend or foe? *World J. Gastroenterol.* **2017**, *23*, 3396–3406. [CrossRef]

93. Moreira de Macêdo, S.; Guimarães, T.A.; Feltenberger, J.D.; Sousa Santos, S.H. The role of renin-angiotensin system modulation on treatment and prevention of liver diseases. *Peptides* **2014**, *62*, 189–196. [CrossRef]

94. Shim, K.Y.; Eom, Y.W.; Kim, M.Y.; Kang, S.H.; Baik, S.K. Role of the renin-angiotensin system in hepatic fibrosis and portal hypertension. *Korean J. Intern. Med.* **2018**, *33*, 453–461. [CrossRef]

95. Mak, K.Y.; Chin, R.; Cunningham, S.C.; Habib, M.R.; Torresi, J.; Sharland, A.F.; Alexander, I.E.; Angus, P.W.; Herath, C.B. ACE2 Therapy Using Adeno-associated Viral Vector Inhibits Liver Fibrosis in Mice. *Mol. Ther.* **2015**, *23*, 1434–1443. [CrossRef]

96. Osterreicher, C.H.; Taura, K.; De Minicis, S.; Seki, E.; Penz-Osterreicher, M.; Kodama, Y.; Kluwe, J.; Schuster, M.; Oudit, G.Y.; Penninger, J.M.; et al. Angiotensin-converting-enzyme 2 inhibits liver fibrosis in mice. *Hepatology* **2009**, *50*, 929–938. [CrossRef] [PubMed]

97. Saldanha da Silva, A.A.; Rodrigues Prestes, T.R.; Lauar, A.O.; Finotti, B.B.; Simoes, E.; Silva, A.C. Renin Angiotensin System and Cytokines in Chronic Kidney Disease: Clinical and Experimental Evidence. *Protein Pept. Lett.* **2017**, *24*, 799–808. [CrossRef]

98. Caruso-Neves, C.; Lara, L.S.; Rangel, L.B.; Grossi, A.L.; Lopes, A.G. Angiotensin-(1–7) modulates the ouabain-insensitive Na+-ATPase activity from basolateral membrane of the proximal tubule. *Biochim. Biophys. Acta* **2000**, *1467*, 189–197. [CrossRef]

99. Lara, L.S.; Bica, R.B.S.; Sena, S.L.F.; Correa, J.S.; Marques-Fernandes, M.F.; Lopes, A.G.; Caruso-Neves, C. Angiotensin-(1–7) reverts the stimulatory effect of angiotensin II on the proximal tubule Na(+)-ATPase activity via a A779-sensitive receptor. *Regul. Pept.* **2002**, *103*, 17–22. [CrossRef]

100. Esteban, V.; Heringer-Walther, S.; Sterner-Kock, A.; de Bruin, R.; van den Engel, S.; Wang, Y.; Mezzano, S.; Egido, J.; Schultheiss, H.-P.; Ruiz-Ortega, M.; et al. Angiotensin-(1–7) and the g protein-coupled receptor MAS are key players in renal inflammation. *PLoS ONE* **2009**, *4*, e5406. [CrossRef]

101. Jiang, T.; Gao, L.; Guo, J.; Lu, J.; Wang, Y.; Zhang, Y. Suppressing inflammation by inhibiting the NF-κB pathway contributes to the neuroprotective effect of angiotensin-(1–7) in rats with permanent cerebral ischaemia. *Br. J. Pharmacol.* **2012**, *167*, 1520–1532. [CrossRef]

102. Chiu, A.T.; Ryan, J.W.; Stewart, J.M.; Dorer, F.E. Formation of angiotensin III by angiotensin-converting enzyme. *Biochem. J.* **1976**, *155*, 189–192. [CrossRef]

103. Cesari, M.; Rossi, G.P.; Pessina, A.C. Biological properties of the angiotensin peptides other than angiotensin II: Implications for hypertension and cardiovascular diseases. *J. Hypertens.* **2002**, *20*, 793–799. [CrossRef]

104. Padia, S.H.; Kemp, B.A.; Howell, N.L.; Siragy, H.M.; Fournie-Zaluski, M.-C.; Roques, B.P.; Carey, R.M. Intrarenal aminopeptidase N inhibition augments natriuretic responses to angiotensin III in angiotensin type 1 receptor-blocked rats. *Hypertension* **2007**, *49*, 625–630. [CrossRef]

105. Kotlo, K.; Hughes, D.E.; Herrera, V.L.M.; Ruiz-Opazo, N.; Costa, R.H.; Robey, R.B.; Danziger, R.S. Functional polymorphism of the Anpep gene increases promoter activity in the Dahl salt-resistant rat. *Hypertension* **2007**, *49*, 467–472. [CrossRef] [PubMed]

106. Carrera, M.P.; Ramírez-Expósito, M.J.; Valenzuela, M.T.; Dueñas, B.; García, M.J.; Mayas, M.D.; Martínez-Martos, J.M. Renin-angiotensin system-regulating aminopeptidase activities are modified in the pineal gland of rats with breast cancer induced by N-methyl-nitrosourea. *Cancer Invest.* **2006**, *24*, 149–153. [CrossRef]

107. Chai, S.Y.; Fernando, R.; Peck, G.; Ye, S.-Y.; Mendelsohn, F.A.O.; Jenkins, T.A.; Albiston, A.L. The angiotensin IV/AT4 receptor. *Cell. Mol. Life Sci.* **2004**, *61*, 2728–2737. [CrossRef] [PubMed]

108. Appenrodt, E.; Brattström, A. Effects of central angiotensin II and angiotensin III on baroreflex regulation. *Neuropeptides* **1994**, *26*, 175–180. [CrossRef]

109. Handa, R.K. Biphasic actions of angiotensin IV on renal blood flow in the rat. *Regul. Pept.* **2006**, *136*, 23–29. [CrossRef] [PubMed]

110. Albiston, A.L.; McDowall, S.G.; Matsacos, D.; Sim, P.; Clune, E.; Mustafa, T.; Lee, J.; Mendelsohn, F.A.; Simpson, R.J.; Connolly, L.M.; et al. Evidence that the angiotensin IV (AT(4)) receptor is the enzyme insulin-regulated aminopeptidase. *J. Biol. Chem.* **2001**, *276*, 48623–48626. [CrossRef] [PubMed]

111. Lochard, N.; Thibault, G.; Silversides, D.W.; Touyz, R.M.; Reudelhuber, T.L. Chronic production of angiotensin IV in the brain leads to hypertension that is reversible with an angiotensin II AT1 receptor antagonist. *Circ. Res.* **2004**, *94*, 1451–1457. [CrossRef]

112. Li, X.C.; Campbell, D.J.; Ohishi, M.; Yuan, S.; Zhuo, J.L. AT1 receptor-activated signaling mediates angiotensin IV-induced renal cortical vasoconstriction in rats. *Am. J. Physiol. Renal Physiol.* **2006**, *290*, F1024–F1033. [CrossRef] [PubMed]

113. Jankowski, V.; Vanholder, R.; van der Giet, M.; Tölle, M.; Karadogan, S.; Gobom, J.; Furkert, J.; Oksche, A.; Krause, E.; Tran, T.N.A.; et al. Mass-spectrometric identification of a novel angiotensin peptide in human plasma. *Arterioscler. Thromb. Vasc. Biol.* **2007**, *27*, 297–302. [CrossRef]

114. Yang, R.; Smolders, I.; Vanderheyden, P.; Demaegdt, H.; Van Eeckhaut, A.; Vauquelin, G.; Lukaszuk, A.; Tourwé, D.; Chai, S.Y.; Albiston, A.L.; et al. Pressor and renal hemodynamic effects of the novel angiotensin A peptide are angiotensin II type 1A receptor dependent. *Hypertension* **2011**, *57*, 956–964. [CrossRef] [PubMed]

115. Coutinho, D.C.O.; Foureaux, G.; Rodrigues, K.D.L.; Salles, R.L.A.; Moraes, P.L.; Murça, T.M.; De Maria, M.L.A.; Gomes, E.R.M.; Santos, R.A.S.; Guatimosim, S.; et al. Cardiovascular effects of angiotensin A: A novel peptide of the renin-angiotensin system. *J. Renin. Angiotensin Aldosterone Syst.* **2014**, *15*, 480–486. [CrossRef] [PubMed]

116. Lautner, R.Q.; Villela, D.C.; Fraga-Silva, R.A.; Silva, N.; Verano-Braga, T.; Costa-Fraga, F.; Jankowski, J.; Jankowski, V.; Sousa, F.; Alzamora, A.; et al. Discovery and characterization of alamandine: A novel component of the renin-angiotensin system. *Circ. Res.* **2013**, *112*, 1104–1111. [CrossRef]

117. Tetzner, A.; Gebolys, K.; Meinert, C.; Klein, S.; Uhlich, A.; Trebicka, J.; Villacañas, Ó.; Walther, T. G-Protein-Coupled Receptor MrgD Is a Receptor for Angiotensin-(1–7) Involving Adenylyl Cyclase, cAMP, and Phosphokinase, A. *Hypertension* **2016**, *68*, 185–194. [CrossRef]

118. Habiyakare, B.; Alsaadon, H.; Mathai, M.L.; Hayes, A.; Zulli, A. Reduction of angiotensin A and alamandine vasoactivity in the rabbit model of atherogenesis: Differential effects of alamandine and Ang(1–7). *Int. J. Exp. Pathol.* **2014**, *95*, 290–295. [CrossRef] [PubMed]

119. Mogielnicki, A.; Kramkowski, K.; Hermanowicz, J.M.; Leszczynska, A.; Przyborowski, K.; Buczko, W. Angiotensin-(1–9) enhances stasis-induced venous thrombosis in the rat because of the impairment of fibrinolysis. *J Renin. Angiotensin Aldosterone Syst.* **2014**, *15*, 13–21. [CrossRef] [PubMed]

120. Karwowska-Polecka, W.; Kułakowska, A.; Wiśniewski, K.; Braszko, J.J. Losartan influences behavioural effects of angiotensin II(3–7) in rats. *Pharmacol. Res.* **1997**, *36*, 275–283. [CrossRef]

121. Handa, R.K. Metabolism alters the selectivity of angiotensin-(1–7) receptor ligands for angiotensin receptors. *J. Am. Soc. Nephrol.* **2000**, *11*, 1377–1386. [PubMed]

122. Nehme, A.; Marcelo, P.; Nasser, R.; Kobeissy, F.; Bricca, G.; Zibara, K. The kinetics of angiotensin-I metabolism in human carotid atheroma: An emerging role for angiotensin (1–7). *Vascul. Pharmacol.* **2016**. [CrossRef] [PubMed]

123. Nehme, A.; Cerutti, C.; Zibara, K. Transcriptomic analysis reveals novel transcription factors associated with renin-angiotensin-aldosterone system in human atheroma. *Hypertension* **2016**, *68*, 1375–1384. [CrossRef]

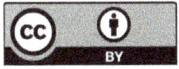

MDPI

St. Alban-Anlage 66

4052 Basel

Switzerland

Tel. +41 61 683 77 34

Fax +41 61 302 89 18

www.mdpi.com

Journal of Cardiovascular Development and Disease Editorial Office

E-mail: jcdd@mdpi.com

www.mdpi.com/journal/jcdd

www.ingramcontent.com/pod-product-compliance
Lightning Source LLC
LaVergne TN
LVHW070544100526
838202LV00012B/374